Making the Right Connections

The design and management
of health care delivery

Making the Right Connections

The design and management of health care delivery

Anthony Harrison

King's Fund

Published by
King's Fund Publishing
11–13 Cavendish Square
London W1G 0AN

First published 2001

ISBN 1 85717 440 2

A CIP catalogue record for this book is available from the British Library

Available from:
King's Fund Bookshop
11–13 Cavendish Square
London
W1G 0AN

Tel: 020 7307 2591
Fax: 020 7307 2801

Typeset by Saxon Graphics Ltd, Derby

Printed and bound in Great Britain

Cover photograph: creativ collection

Contents

Foreword and acknowledgements

In January 2000, Jennifer Dixon and I published *The NHS: Facing the Future*,[1] a wide-ranging overview that identified a number of long-standing weaknesses in the NHS. Three of these – its persistent inability to get the right organisational structure, the design of services and the ineffectual link between workforce and service planning – form the focus of this book.

Many of the ideas that are set out below, however, come from work with my former colleague Seán Boyle when he led the King's Fund team supporting the second King's Fund London Commission. Out of that collaboration came a series of papers, some of which remain unpublished,[2] that explored the notion of health care delivery as a *system*. Other King's Fund colleagues were thinking along similar lines but using quite different approaches.[3]

It would be hard to establish who was first to apply the notion of a *system* to the delivery of health care. As far as back as 1971, however, Paul Sanazaro set out to describe the development of the hospital in the context of 'health services systems'.[4] His central historical perception was that:

> *... hospital services are on a plateau in their evolution while health services and their contributing sciences are in transition towards more formal systems. Leading up to the plateau are centuries of unco-ordinated, autonomous growth. Ahead is the era of interdependent planning and decision-making which will integrate all institutional and extra-institutional health services.* (p 132)

In fact his expectations proved over-optimistic. The hoped-for integration is still being sought. But his central notion that

> *The system concept imposes the requirement to bring about and maintain functional relationships among existing components so as to assure performance in accord with specified criteria.* (p 141)

has at last been recognised. The term 'system' is now widely in use, in both official and professional papers,[5] but it is rarely defined. Two definitions may be helpful. One comes from a study of international politics:

> *We are dealing with a system when (a) a set of ... elements is interconnected so that changes in some elements or their relations produce changes in other parts of the system, and (b) the entire system exhibits properties and behaviours that are different from those of the parts.*[6]

The second comes from a study of primary care in the NHS:

> *A system is defined as a number of interactive elements which together make up a defined whole; analysis is concerned with how the whole system relates to its environment and how the elements within the system interact in doing so.*[7]

These definitions embrace the main ideas with which we shall be concerned in this book: the notions of interconnection and interaction between elements that are apparently distinct, but which can beneficially be regarded as parts of a greater whole.

While the system notion is coming into general use in official and professional papers, the task of getting the functional relationships among existing elements – the organisations and professions that make up a health service and the rules under which they operate – remains. But these 'existing elements' are not necessarily the right ones. They exist now as a result of historical processes that took little or no account of the system concept.

That history cannot be discarded; we are where we are. But for part of what follows we pretend that it can, by indulging in a thought experiment: if we were to design a care delivery system from scratch, how would we go about it?

To answer this apparently simple question, this book must, like *The NHS: Facing the Future*, take a helicopter view of a vast terrain, made even more forbidding by the absence of a co-pilot, and too wide to map through systematic review. The aim, therefore, has been to keep references in the text to a modest level and to provide, through footnotes, signposts to the much wider literature on which it draws.

This text has benefited from comments from my colleagues in the Health Systems programme – John Appleby, Justin Keen and Jo-Ann Mulligan. I am also grateful to Shirley Harrison, Kim Stirling, Trevor Anderson and Mandy Howard for their help in preparing the text for publication and to Lucy Johnson for literature searches, and to her and all her colleagues in the King's Fund Library and Information Service for their support throughout the project.

AJH
King's Fund
November 2000

References

1. Harrison and Dixon, 2000.
2. These papers include *Why waiting lists grow* and *Modelling urgent events*. They are available from AJH.
3. See Pratt *et al.*, 1999.
4. See Sanazaro, 1971. Sanazaro was at the time Director of the National Center for Health Services Research and Development in Washington, DC. In an earlier Nuffield paper, Brotherston had referred to 'the medicare-care systems of all advanced countries'. In recent years the term has been taken up by more authors than can be mentioned here.
5. Examples are given in later chapters. Perhaps the most striking use of the term by a politician was that of the Secretary of State for Health, Alan Milburn, in a speech to the year 2000 conference of the NHS Confederation, when he asserted that the NHS was neither a market nor a hierarchy but a system. It appeared not to have occurred to his speechwriters that both markets and hierarchies might also be considered systems. See also Exworthy, Powell and Mohan, 1999, who correctly argue that the NHS has co-existing elements of market, hierarchy and network.
6. Jervis, 1997, p 6.
7. Boaden, 1997, p 57.

PART ONE

Policy development

Chapter One

Introduction

What would NHS care be like in an ideal world? Although opinions will vary, most would consider that it should provide high quality care that is readily accessible, in terms of time and distance, and that the professionals providing the care treat their patients with respect and keep them informed of what is happening to them and of the implications of alternative courses of treatment. Where care involves contributions from more than one professional, the links between those contributions should be effectively made from initial contact through to final outcome.[1]

But, while it is easy enough to set out the general characteristics of the ideal health care service, it is much harder to define how services should be provided on the ground such that the chances of those characteristics being realised are maximised. Even in a world where resources were unlimited, difficult choices would have to be made. For example, the best quality may be obtainable only at the cost of reduced access. Such tensions between quality and access have to be faced in *any* health care system, however well resourced, though geographical factors and the available finance will lead to different resolutions of those tensions in different countries or in different parts of the same country. As long as people require facilities of the kind currently found in hospitals, which can only be provided effectively in clinical terms if they serve large catchment areas, that will be true.

In the real world, the cost of different ways of providing services also has to be taken into account. From the viewpoint of those funding health care services – the Treasury in the case of the NHS – the key requirement of a health care delivery system is that services are delivered efficiently and effectively and that the total cost of doing so is kept under control. While easy access may be a goal for the individual, for the system as a whole control of access is a necessity for cost containment.[2] It follows that, though health care is or should be focused on the individual seeking care, the design of the Service must be carried out with an eye to other considerations.

The choice between different locations for health care delivery would form a major area of concern in the design of an ideal health care system, but many other issues would also have to be resolved; for example:

- the balance between specialists and generalists
- the number of hospital specialties there should be
- whether everyone should have his or her own GP
- how the 'work' required in delivering care should be divided between different professional groups
- whether GPs should gatekeep for all other health care services or, if not for all, for which
- whether hospital services should form part of one organisation and community-based services another.

The answers to some of these issues have been largely taken for granted (of course people should have their own GP) or ignored (there is no explicit policy or public debate about the total number of specialties). Others, such as the balance between specialists and generalists and the boundaries between professions, are debated in the professional journals but, for the most part, these issues have attracted only modest attention from researchers and policy-makers. And, where they have been considered, they have been considered individually, rather than as a set of related issues bearing on the structure of the Service as a whole.

These issues can be rephrased into a series of simple questions: which elements should a service consist of, who should provide them, in which locations, by what size and coverage of organisation, and how should these various elements combine with each other? The way in which these apparently simple questions are answered will determine the structure of the Service.[3]

Over the life of the NHS, these issues have never been systematically addressed. The structure of the NHS, like that of other health care systems, reflects the accidents of history as much as the intentions of policy-makers. The division of roles between hospital and community staff reflects both the nature of the political settlement which made the NHS possible and the structure of medical care that had emerged over the previous 50 years. The NHS did not start with a blank slate and design itself from scratch: it was largely built around structures that had emerged as a result of professional rivalries on the one hand and the unsystematic and unco-ordinated attempts of local authorities and charitable organisations to provide hospital services on the other. Differences in structure at local level were not ironed out so as to ensure that the NHS delivered care in a uniform way across the country as a whole.

In fact, a blueprint was to hand: more than 20 years before, a committee under the chairmanship of Lord Dawson, a leading physician of his day, had set out a vision of how health care delivery should be structured.[4] But although the Dawson report was re-published by the King's Fund in 1950 because of its continuing relevance, it continued to be ignored. Since then no similar report has emerged from the national level of the NHS or from any other government body, covering, in one document, all the elements that define how care is delivered.[5]

Design failure

Despite this apparent lack of interest, ever since its foundation both policy-makers and clinicians have been concerned about the structure of the Service. Much of that concern has been focused on the question of how the various parts of the Service should work together and what the appropriate administrative structure should be to ensure that they do.

The need to overcome the many barriers that prevent effective working between different parts of the NHS was reflected in official documents from the 1950s, such as the Guillebaud report,[6] in the major structural reforms in the 1970s when local government health services were transferred to central government control, and to the Labour Government's proposals in *The New NHS*[7] published in 1997.

The importance of financial and other barriers within the NHS emerged strongly when, in the 1990s, the notion took hold that services could generally be moved from hospital to community settings. But the division between finance for hospitals and finance for general medical services made that difficult; if care was shifted, finance did not follow.[8] As a result, the 'best' balance between hospital and community could not emerge.[9]

Gradually, however, the emphasis has shifted from changes in administrative structures to the delivery of care itself. From the 1980s onwards, the need to ensure the harmonious working of the various parts of the NHS was highlighted by changes within hospitals. A combination of financial pressures and changes in clinical technology led to ever shorter lengths of stay and a withdrawal from long-term care for elderly people. This switch had been facilitated during the early 1990s by the ready availability of nursing home beds financed out of social security funds. When that 'escape route' was closed by the transfer of these funds to local authorities, the result was the emergence of bed blocking. Local authorities were often slow to take on responsibility for patients when they were ready for discharge from hospital, while hospital management proved unequal to the task of discharging the ever-larger number of patients passing through them.

The resulting failures were well documented in a series of reports from the Clinical Standards Advisory Group[10] and from the Audit Commission,[11] as well as academic investigators. They also revealed, however, that not only did services for groups such as elderly people fail to mesh properly together but also that the NHS lacked some of the basic skills to design and deliver services to ensure that they did. The weaknesses revealed, in other words, stemmed not simply from barriers to collaborative working arising from administrative structures or financial rules, but also from an inability to design services properly, i.e. to identify who should do what and how the links between the various elements required for effective care could best be made.

Such weaknesses were found in major services. In 1979, for example, a study of stroke care[12] found that:

> *Current provisions of health and community services differ for each health district. The services provided are the product of haphazard and irregular growth in response to the interests of health care professionals, philanthropists, social reformers, and local pressure groups. Demand rather than need has often dominated decision-making on service provision.* (p 51)

More than 20 years later, an overview of stroke care in the UK[13] and other parts of Europe reported that:

> *Studies in Europe and surveys from The Stroke Association indicate that service provision is still haphazard, fragmented and often sub-optimal. Although the efficacy of many of the interventions may be unclear, there is current geographical inequality in the services that stroke patients receive. The current overall pattern of services cannot be cost-effective.* (p 5)

Towards the end of the 1990s, the most overt sign of failure was the series of winter crises that seemed to afflict the Service on an annual basis. The Service had already tried to respond to winter pressures by co-ordinating action across both hospital and community services. These efforts[14] led to the identification of a large number of proposals for improving performance, but there was no systematic analysis of the factors at work or of the reasons why performance was poor.

Recognising the need for a more fundamental review, in 1998 the then Secretary of State, Frank Dobson, commissioned from his department a National Beds Inquiry, which eventually reported in February 2000 – the first report on hospital services as a whole from the Centre[15] for 20 years. This, however, did not set out a clear vision of the future: rather, it emphasised the uncertainties facing the future of hospitals and the large number of issues that had to be resolved before a clear view of their role in the health care system as a whole could emerge. Similarly, reports on intensive care facilities from the Audit Commission[16] and an expert group[17] found that little systematic attention had been paid to their adequacy or their effective management within the hospital as a whole. Subsequently, the Government announced proposals in the NHS Plan[18] for developing intermediate care facilities.

The same lack of design capacity was apparent for the hospital sector as a whole. How all these elements were to fit together was left to health authorities, who had little capacity for work of this kind. The NHS spent a great deal of effort during the 1960s in trying to establish how hospital services ought to be delivered. Both the 1962 Hospital Plan[19] and the Bonham Carter report [20] seven years later aimed to define the proper role of the hospital, what its scale and scope should be, and how the respective roles of the hospital and the community should be defined. But in the 1970s the issues were generally neglected.

During the 1980s and 1990s, however, concern about the structure of the Service and the organisation of clinical work within it began to emerge through professional reports on emergency services[21] and the reviews carried out in London for the London Implementation Group.[22] The emphasis in these reports was on the structure and scale of particular hospital specialties. In the case of cancer, a national-level expert committee[23] was subsequently established. This produced recommendations in 1995 for the structure of cancer services as a whole, which were designed to overcome what appeared to be the poor performance of the NHS when measured against other countries. Its primary criticism was that cancer care was insufficiently specialised: hospital structures developed to provide accessible local services were inappropriate for modern cancer care.[24]

The Labour Government's White Paper, *The New NHS*,[25] took up this theme with its proposals for national service frameworks. These aim to work out how to provide a service for a large group of patients, taking all forms of provision into account. By 2000, the first results of this new process were emerging in the form of a series of recommendations bearing on the design and delivery of care for coronary heart disease and mental illness, and also a National Cancer Plan that built on and expanded the proposals of the expert committee. These developments, however, took place on a service-by-service basis: the 'whole system' of which they formed part remained neglected.

There was a parallel but different development within community-based services. Towards the end of its period of office, the Conservative Government published two White Papers on primary care and followed these up with the 1999 Primary Care Act. This led to a large number of local experiments with different ways of providing services in the community, which in effect acknowledged that the NHS could not continue to rely solely on the traditional way of providing medical services. Furthermore, the new Labour Government introduced two new policies – NHS Direct[26] and walk-in centres – that were designed to make services more accessible to users but which appeared to undermine general practice, the existing means of delivering medical services in the community, by offering people an alternative source of first contact care. As with the service frameworks, these developments appeared piecemeal. Although they formed part of the Government's overall strategy to make the NHS more 'patient centred', how the services on the ground should relate to each other, if at all, remained unclear.

Workforce skills

While these developments were occurring at service level, parallel changes were taking place in the workforce. The present structure of the NHS's workforce – the definition of each of the professions and the roles they play in the delivery of care – can be explained only by their historical development over the last two centuries. The resulting 'balkanisation' of the workforce into professions, specialties and sub-specialties produced a situation, typical of much of the British manufacturing industry up to the 1980s, where changes of role were virtually impossible and relationships between professional groups were poor or non-existent. For the patient, it meant that the care journey was fractured: for the Service, it meant that services fitted into professional roles rather than the reverse.

The need to tackle professional boundaries and barriers was recognised in the 1990s in a series of initiatives by the professions, such as the joint statement between the medical and nursing professions on collaborative working.[27] A number of local or small-scale developments began to break down the barriers between professions, including the introduction of nurse practitioners and nurse prescribing, the partial replacement of junior doctors with specialist nurses, and other attempts at role substitution such as generic workers. In hospitals and general practice, team working involving a range of professions and skills became common. In 1997, the Institute of Health Service Managers published a report[28] on the future NHS workforce, which put forward a series of radical ideas for the redesign of professional roles. Work for the North Thames Region of the NHS[29] revealed the complexity of making changes of that kind: it found that over 60 organisations and types of organisation were involved in the development of the workforce and most had little connection with service design or delivery. It was unsurprising, therefore, that the links between workforce and service planning were poor.

In 1999, the Health Select Committee of the House of Commons published a highly critical report of workforce planning[30] that took up this issue. It found that the training of the workforce was effectively detached from the day-to-day process of services delivery, but it nevertheless had a profound influence upon it. Thus, change in the structure of hospital services, particularly the trend towards larger hospitals, largely reflected changes within the medical workforce, particularly its training requirements and the growth of specialisation. This central issue – failure to link workforce and service planning – was recognised in the Government's response to the Select Committee.[31] This acknowledged the need for a fundamental review, the first results of which were published in April 2000.[32] However, though that made a number of radical proposals, it failed to suggest how service delivery and training could be more effectively linked. That task remains.

Enduring weaknesses

The weaknesses briefly described above may come as a surprise to those from other health care systems. From the outside, the fact that the NHS works under common rules of finance and ownership has seemed to ensure it would possess an ideal structure for effective service delivery. As the evidence from external audits of the Service carried out by the Audit Commission and the Clinical Standards Advisory Group during the 1990s showed, in practice these general features did little to ensure the various parts of the NHS worked well together or to counteract the forces making for balkanisation between professions. And so we find in Labour's White Paper, *The New NHS*, published 50 years after the foundation of the NHS, terms such as 'partnership', 'joint working', 'co-operation' and so on, which by their very presence in the document indicated the failure of previous attempts to counter these forces. The White Paper put part of the blame for the 'disintegration' of the Service on the previous government's attempts to introduce competition. But, while there is some justification for this charge, it overlooks the fact that the Service had failed to design and provide integrated services prior to 1991. However, the administrative and financial changes the White Paper proposed,[33] later enacted in the 1999 Health Act, meant that some of the remaining structural barriers were removed or reduced. Furthermore, the national service frameworks and other policies looked at in more detail below suggested that issues of service design were at last being tackled.

But while these developments are overdue and hence welcome now, they suffer from several weaknesses.

First, the connections between them have not been properly made. Even though government documents use the term 'whole systems',[34] none attempts to take into account the health care delivery system as a whole. There is no one place, nor has there ever been, where all the elements of the NHS structure are considered at one and the same time. Furthermore, even now some of the central structural features of the NHS, particularly the role of the medical workforce, remain largely unchallenged.

The role of the GP as gatekeeper, the virtual elimination of the GP from the hospital and the virtual identification of the hospital with specialist care, are key defining elements of the British NHS. So too are the rules, some backed by statute, others more by convention, that govern the roles of different members of the workforce. Despite the fact that the way training is organised and the Service is divided between specialties is so central to the way that health care services are delivered, how decisions are reached on these issues is almost invisible – and hence they receive very little systematic scrutiny as to their impact and value. As we have noted elsewhere,[35] the Royal Colleges have been a 'state within a state', accountable to none but themselves, but having a large impact on the way the Service works.

Second, most of these new policy developments take the existing framework of professional roles for granted and do not consider other possibilities. The NHS was built round the separation between community and hospital doctors, but other countries do not draw the line in the same way. In many, specialists who would be found only in hospitals in the UK are available in the community. Similarly, while the UK ambulance services cover transport and the relatively limited roles of paramedics, others combine ambulance services with the

delivery of social and health care services. And whil
of their few health rights, the right to register wi
normal point of first contact, other systems run ser
particular groups of the population such children
Options such as merging the roles of communi
others that will emerge later in this book – dc
But, as we shall see, throughout the life of the NHS the
often senior clinicians, who have argued against the grain of the
very different ways of structuring services.

Third, there is no agreed framework, either of concepts or of terminology, for analysing the structure of health care delivery. As things stand, any description of how services are delivered relies on terms that are typically confusing and which do not reflect the changes described above. Counting units, such as the hospital bed or hospital spell, remains in widespread use, despite the fact that changes in the way that health care is actually provided have rendered their simple total an irrelevance.

Nevertheless, in the UK and other countries, new terms are coming into use, such as 'care pathways', 'systems of care', 'disease management' and 'whole systems' which, as argued below, offer much better ways of analysing health care delivery systems. At the same time, there is growing interest in rethinking professional roles and the relationship between the formal organisations that make up the NHS and the services they deliver. But, though these developments are linked, they have taken place without much apparent mutual contact. The main aim of this book is to link together these various strands.

A related aim is to introduce an approach and a language that will abstract from specific national organisations[36] and institutions. To do this we make use of terms – 'routing', 'service design', 'systems of care' – that are just creeping into general use. We make as little use as possible of those familiar terms – 'hospital' and 'primary care' – that have no clear meaning but which, despite their lack of clarity, continue to be used for lack of any obvious alternative.

The issues considered here are common to all countries. Every health care system struggles to balance the need to contain spending with the desire to raise quality. In the First World, all health care systems are experiencing changes in the balance of the needs they serve towards chronic disease and other conditions associated with old age. All are faced with rapidly changing medical and related technologies. All are faced with increasingly knowledgeable users, as information of a kind once available only to professionals becomes widely available.

ough there is a vast comparative literature comparing health care s, much of it sheds little light on the 'real' health economy, i.e. the health ices themselves. Instead, the literature largely focuses on funding systems d the pattern of ownership. Although health care is produced in different ways, much of the technology – drugs, surgical procedures, etc. – is common. But the history of each country and its set of institutions are different so, rather like national economies, they work slightly differently even if the underlying technology and knowledge base are similar. Some differences can be seen at a superficial level, e.g. the ratio of doctors to nurses varies widely in western Europe, but others, such as the nature of the links between hospital and community-based services, are often hard to disentangle.

This book

As we show in the first part of this book, over the years the NHS has been reorganised on several occasions, with the aim of providing a more effective and efficient structure. These reorganisations did not bear directly on the way that services themselves were provided but more on the structure of the supervisory layer – the districts and regions that come between local service delivery and the Centre. Only recently have new initiatives emerged, such as national service frameworks and primary care act pilots, which do bear directly on service provision.

Building on a series of recent developments, the second part of this book sets out an analytic framework that we argue can be used to describe health care delivery systems in a new way. We then focus first on service users and then on the professionals providing care, with the aim of bringing out the implications for each of this new approach.

Next, we consider some of the issues that accompany the new approach, taking first the new set of technical issues they raise and then their relationship with existing institutions. We find that current forms of organisation must be adapted to the new requirements of effective service delivery. The present structure of accountability within the NHS, including its external audit, is targeted on organisations, not on services and whole systems. Training and research continue to be focused on the specific skill rather than the care system. As shown below, many of the areas that are critical to the working of whole care systems continue to be ignored in the professional literature. Finally, the new performance management arrangements now being introduced for the NHS and social care reflect only in a very modest degree the changes that have already been made in the development of systems of care.

We conclude with a brief review of the current situation. Our main finding is that thinking about health care delivery is moving in the right direction, away from a preoccupation with the specific clinical intervention towards systems of care. But the new approaches have not yet been thought through. As a result, a large technical and policy agenda remains.

References

1. This paragraph is not intended to be exhaustive of the characteristics users value in health care delivery. Other aspects will be considered in Chapter Six.
2. This sentence reflects the UK experience of a low-spending health service but nevertheless applies to better-resourced systems.
3. By 'structure' we refer to the organisation of the Service as a whole – including its administrative framework, the organisation of broad groups of services such as hospitals (i.e. their financial and accountability framework), the division of the workforce into groupings such as professions and specialties, and the rules, such as the gatekeeping role of GPs, which determine how the various elements relate to each other.
4. Dawson, 1920, reprinted 1950.
5. The NHS Plan, though a wide-ranging document, has nothing to say about, for example, emergency care or hospitals as a whole.
6. Guillebaud, 1956.
7. Secretary of State for Health, 1997
8. Many schemes promoting transfer were funded by non-recurring monies: once these ran out, they were often abandoned.
9. Cultural factors also played a large part in frustrating change, particularly the long-standing divide between hospital-based doctors and those working in the community.
10. Clinical Standards Advisory Group, 1998.
11. Audit Commission, 1995.
12. Weddell and Beresford, 1979.
13. Wolfe *et al.*, 1997.
14. NHS Executive, 2000a
15. Department of Health, 2000g. We use the term 'Centre' to refer to the Department of Health (and its predecessors, the Ministry of Health and the Department of Health and Social Security) and the NHS Executive (and its predecessor, the NHS Management Executive).
16. Audit Commission, 1999a.
17. Department of Health, 2000b.
18. Secretary of State for Health, 2000.
19. Ministry of Health, 1962.
20. Ministry of Health, 1969.
21. See, for example, Royal College of Surgeons, 1997, 2000.
22. London Implementation Group, 1993.

23. Always known as Calman/Hine after its joint chairs.
24. Department of Health and Welsh Office, 1995.
25. Secretary of State for Health, 1997.
26. NHS Direct is a telephone advice service. Begun on a pilot basis in 1998, it is now a national system.
27. Standing Medical and Nursing & Midwifery Advisory Committees, 1996.
28. Health Services Management Unit, 1996.
29. NHS Executive North Thames, 1997a & b.
30. House of Commons, 1999a & b.
31. Department of Health, 1999c.
32. Department of Health, 2000d.
33. The changes included the merger of finance for hospital and nearly all community-based services.
34. See, for example, Department of Health and NHS Executive, 1998a.
35. Harrison and Prentice, 1996.
36. The term 'organisation' is itself highly ambiguous. In much of what follows, we examine the tension between organisations with a clear accountability structure, such as UK trusts and GP practices, with organised systems of care based largely on clinical practices, sometimes formalised in protocols, sometimes simply reflecting accepted routines, which do not have – at least at present – a distinct formal organisation complete with financial and other accounting requirements but which are organised in the sense that they work according to a set of clinical conventions that are stable and understood among those within the system of care.

Chapter Two

The search for the right structure

For most of its life, the NHS has been in a state of continuous administrative revolution. As we shall see in the first part of this chapter, the links between such change and expected improvement in service delivery were rarely made clear, but from the 1950s onwards, change in administrative structures has been seen as vital to the effective development and delivery of services across the various elements the NHS comprises – hospital, general practice and community health services.

Nevertheless, despite what have been fundamental administrative changes, at no time since its foundation has the NHS attempted to define what pattern of services it should deliver. Instead, a series of initiatives has been taken that bears on particular services such as hospitals, on professional roles such as changes to the GP contract, or on the organisations responsible for providing care such as NHS trusts. The overall structure, as it now stands, therefore, is the result of piecemeal and partial developments rather than a comprehensive attempt to define how the NHS should deliver care. This chapter considers some of the most important of these developments:

- the administrative structure of the Service
- the broad balance of care between hospitals and community-based services
- the whole system
- the structure of the workforce
- the role of users.

In the final section of the chapter, we identify a number of key themes that have emerged from this piecemeal development and which point the way towards a systematic approach.

Administrative structure

From almost its earliest days, the NHS was conscious that its organisational structure did not match the needs of service delivery. Reflecting the political struggle over its formation, the Service that emerged in 1948 was split into three main divisions: a hospital service (itself divided into two parts); general practice; and community health services under the control of local authorities.

In 1955, when the Guillebaud Committee of Enquiry into the Cost of the NHS published its report,[1] it concluded that these divisions were undesirable.

> *113. Many people, both before and after the Appointed Day, have criticised the tripartite structure of the National Health Service because of*
>
> a) *the difficulty of integrating the service provided by the three branches of the National Health Service, particularly in relation to the maternity and child welfare, tuberculosis, mental and aged sick services;*
> b) *the danger of duplication and overlapping between the three branches of the Service;*
> c) *the difficulty of adjusting priorities within the Health Service, when three separate administrative organisations – two financed wholly by the Exchequer and the third partly by the Exchequer and partly by the local rates – are responsible for the provision of the services;*
> d) *the danger that the Service may develop into a National* Hospital *Service, with all the emphasis on curative medicine, instead of a National* Health *Service in which prevention will play as important a part as cure.* (p 54)[2]

As this extract shows, the structural weaknesses were seen in broad terms rather than in terms of specific failings. The implicit assumption was that if the weaknesses in organisational structure were removed, the hoped-for integration of services for children and for elderly and mentally ill people would be achieved.

During the 1960s and early 1970s, a series of Green and White Papers on the administrative structure of the NHS came to similar conclusions.[3] The result was the 1974 reorganisation that succeeded in bringing all the elements of the NHS into one administrative structure presided over by the DHSS. But within that it created a bipartite rather than a unified service: while hospital and community services came within one chain of command, general practice remained apart.

The first and only Royal Commission on the NHS was appointed in 1976 and reported three years later.[4] The Government accepted the Commission's recommendation that regional health authorities and district health authorities should be introduced, but the administrative structure of the NHS at ground level still remained divided between the two main branches of the Service.

After a number of further changes, administrative merger of the NHS supervisory apparatus was eventually achieved in 1995 with the creation of unified district health authorities responsible for hospital and all community-based services including general practice.

By that time, however, the 1991 reforms had introduced a new form of organisation – the NHS trust – with new responsibilities for the delivery of services themselves. In many cases, hospital and community-based services were established in separate trusts, whereas before they had been within the same organisations. Health authorities became responsible for the purchasing of care from them. But some of the purchasing role was dispersed to general practice fundholders.[5]

These changes introduced new divisions (between purchasing and providing) and strengthened old ones (between hospital and community). However, the view from the Centre was that the new arrangements would promote effective working across the newly created boundaries. The NHS Management Executive envisaged that the contracting process introduced in the 1991 reforms could be used as an integrating device, i.e. that contracts would replace administrative structures as the integrating agent.[6] In June 1991, it published a paper, *Integrating Primary and Secondary Care*,[7] which contained a series of proposals designed to promote 'the active pursuit of high quality, seamless care at every level across the primary and secondary arms of the service'.

In fact, the notion that contracts might be service integrators was tried out by a small number of trusts for services such as paediatric or elderly care, where the links between hospital and community are, or should be, strong. But it did not become the norm. This failure reflected a wider failure of the contracting process to assert itself over providers. Even where, as in the total purchasing pilots,[8] clinicians were 'in charge', the contracting process does not appear to have been widely used to promote integration of services across organisational boundaries. Thus, by the time the Conservatives left office in 1997, administrative unification of the supervisory apparatus had been achieved, but the hoped-for integration of services across organisational and other boundaries through contracting had not.[9]

Labour's first White Paper argued that the internal market had 'ended up fragmenting decision-making and distorting incentives to such an extent that unfairness and bureaucracy became its defining features' (para 10).[10] In its place, it set out a large range of measures designed to bring the various elements of the NHS into a closer and more effective relationship, which included a duty of partnership within the NHS and between the NHS and local authorities:

> 6.6 *The Government will establish a new statutory duty for NHS Trusts to work in partnership with other NHS organisations. The duty of partnership will require their participation (alongside Primary Care Groups, universities and Local Authorities) in developing the Health Improvement Programme under the leadership of the Health Authority. In turn, the Health Improvement Programme will set the framework for the services NHS Trusts provide and the detailed agreements they make with Primary Care Groups.* (p 45)

The duty of partnership was formally implemented by the 1999 Health Act. The 1999 Act took the important further step of putting virtually all the health finance flowing directly to local purchasers into a single pot,[11] while at the same time creating provisions for some finance to be pooled and used jointly by health and local social service authorities. In this way, it was hoped that some of the financial barriers between the two would be reduced.

Although apparently a new departure, in essence these measures represent a continuation of the earlier tradition of trying to integrate services using administrative measures. At the time of writing, there is little evidence to show that these new measures have proved more effective than those already tried.

The balance of services

Soon after the First World War, the Dawson report already referred to in Chapter One[12] set out a pattern of service delivery based on three groupings: primary health care centres, secondary health care centres and teaching hospitals.

In the event, the Dawson report had little influence on the pattern of services on the ground. By the time the NHS was established, primary care and the hospital service were, in the opinion of contemporary observers, poorly structured for effective service delivery. The notion of the health centre, central to the report's recommendations for both primary and secondary care, was generally disregarded.[13]

The 1962 Hospital Plan[14] was the NHS's first attempt to put in place an appropriate set of services in all parts of the country. Following various reports before and during the Second World War, it was recognised that the NHS's hospitals needed complete restructuring.

The Plan was based on the concept of a district general hospital in each locality, supported by specialist centres on the one hand and local small hospitals on the other. The Plan was subsequently modified in a number of ways, but the central concept that every district should have its own hospital, serving the majority of its needs, remained.

Despite its central place in the health care system, the acute hospital attracted virtually no attention from policy-makers during the 1970s. In 1980, a consultation document[15] on the structure of hospital services was published, but there was no follow-up in the form of a revised plan or set of guidelines. The regional health authorities did have a significant role in shaping hospital services during the 1980s but it was not until 20 years later, with the publication of the National Beds Inquiry in 2000,[16] that the Centre made a substantial contribution, and that, as we shall see, was a limited one.

This neglect of service delivery was apparent in community-based services as well. There was no equivalent to the 1962 Plan for primary care. In 1986, a Blue Paper[17] acknowledged that it represented the first attempt since the foundation of the NHS to review the role of general practice.[18]

Thus, by the time the 1990 reforms were being implemented, the structure of service delivery had received very little attention from national policymakers. Even the Royal Commission, which did consider all parts of the Service, did not ask searching questions about the appropriate size structure and organisation of hospitals or the overall balance between these and community services. The 1990 reforms themselves ignored these issues. Trusts were created largely around existing administrative structures; their continuing appropriateness to the delivery of care received very little attention.[19]

Nevertheless, there was a series of developments during the 1990s bearing on the structure and balance of services, which did not result directly from the 1990 reforms themselves but which have nevertheless proved very important. These concerned:

- the structure of the hospital sector – the size and number of hospitals
- the shift of care from hospital to community
- innovation in general medical services – i.e. new ways of providing the services associated with general practice
- the design of care for specific needs.

We look at these in turn.

Hospital structure

Within the hospital sector, the question of structure and balance was raised by the Tomlinson inquiry[20] into health services in London and the subsequent reports on specialist services by the London Implementation Group (LIG) studies. These all concluded that structural changes were required to provide more effective care.

Their recommendations, like those of the subsequently appointed cancer expert committee,[21] were based on two main considerations: that existing services were insufficiently specialised; and that the nature of the service should be defined across all the relevant providers, from community-based services to the most specialised hospital care.

The pressures for more and larger specialised units were not confined to specialised services. They were particularly strong in the field of accident and emergency services, where proposals were put forward by professionals and others[22] for a small number of 'super' hospitals – as few as 50 for the whole of the UK – each of which would contain the full range of medical and surgical specialties. Although these specific proposals were not implemented, the number of hospitals offering accident and emergency services was progressively reduced during the 1990s.[23]

The second important theme within the LIG studies and the Calman/Hine proposals was the need to consider the whole spectrum of contributions to care and the relationships between hospitals as well as between the hospital and community-based services. The report on plastics and burns,[24] for example, set out a vision of a three-tier service, with the second and third (hospital) tiers divided as between hubs (offering comprehensive services) and spokes (offering day case and outpatient services).

This theme was developed in subsequent official reports. In 1997, the Standing Medical Advisory Group (SMAC)[25] argued for what it termed 'clinical systems of care', which it described as follows:

> 3.2 … *A clinical system of care is an organisation of clinical resources providing care to a clinical group of patients representing the best balance between clinical and cost effectiveness and accessibility.* A *system of care is not*

necessarily limited by current management boundaries nor by physical structures. The optimum size of population served by a system of care may vary for different patient groups and for different medical specialties.

In Scotland, a different language was being developed for essentially similar requirements: the 'managed clinical network'. As with the hub and spoke, one of the motivating factors was the lack of fit between service needs and the size of acute hospitals. The Acute Services Review[26] argued, like SMAC, that:

> 93. *Health care services are delivered across a spectrum of primary, secondary, tertiary and community care. The Review has recognised from the outset that it was quite inappropriate to regard acute services as the exclusive concern of secondary or tertiary hospital services. Significantly, the Review was not constrained by existing boundaries between primary, secondary and tertiary care...* (p 39)

It went on to propose that managed clinical networks[27] should be developed, linking clinicians working in different hospitals but treating similar patient groups. In 2000, NHS Wales published *Access and Excellence*,[28] which also concluded that acute hospital services should be planned beyond the existing boundaries of health authorities and trusts.

The notion of systems of care running across organisational boundaries represents a major change in thinking about service delivery. It undermines the importance of particular institutions such as hospitals and particular roles such as general practice.[29] It will form the basis for much of the analysis in later chapters.

The shift to the community

By a process that in retrospect is not entirely clear, new phrases came into general use in the 1990s, phrases that remained ill-defined but which implied that the balance of services should shift away from hospitals to community settings. In 1989, for example, the King's Fund published *Hospital at Home: The Coming Revolution*[30] and, in the follow-up to the Tomlinson inquiry report, which supported such a shift, a large number of hospital at home projects were established.

At this time, the message was that the balance of the Service could be and should be changed away from hospitals and, more radically, that the balance of power within it should change as well. Terms such as 'the primary care-led

NHS', 'the strategic switch to the community', 'shifting the boundaries' and 'closer to home'[31] came into common use.

Although these terms were seldom precisely defined, their adoption reflected a recognition – more correctly, a re-recognition since the point is clear in Dawson and the 1962 Plan – that the boundaries between hospital and community were not immutable and that technical change had opened the way for care being transferred from one to the other.

But that shift proved hard to achieve. In part this could be put down to the financial barriers already referred to. Where successful transfer schemes were established, they were often wound up once project funding was withdrawn. Nevertheless, these developments began to break down the barriers between hospital and community.

From the mid-1990s, a further impetus became apparent as the NHS gradually came to terms with the bed reductions in acute hospitals that had been taking place as a result of financial and other pressures. These led to renewed interest, in the NHS Plan and other official papers,[32] in the role of community-based facilities (often termed 'intermediate facilities') for reducing the workload of the hospital.

While the notion has gained general acceptance and a number of schemes have been implemented locally, the report of the National Beds Inquiry[33] made it clear that the process for getting the balance between hospital and community facilities right, even for emergency medical admissions, is far from clear. That report declined to offer a clear view of the future but instead put forward a number of scenarios for consultation about the role of the hospital and the balance between its facilities and those in the community. By doing so, it served to emphasise the fluidity of their respective roles and the extent to which they interact with each other. As a result it opened the way for considering the design of services across the hospital–community divide. It did not itself take the opportunity to do so.

Innovation in general medical services

As far as primary care was concerned, the main thrust of the reforms was at the development of its purchasing role rather than provision. In the late 1990s, however, the then Minister for Health conducted a listening exercise that came to the conclusion that the existing administrative framework was too restrictive and held back service improvements.

The subsequent White Papers[34] proposed a series of measures designed to allow forms of service to develop. In their last legislative action, the Conservatives passed the 1997 Act, which opened the way for pilots of new forms of service delivery, an opportunity that the new Labour Government took. The result was a large number of small-scale pilot schemes.

These pilots focused largely on promoting access for groups not well served by the existing form of service delivery such, as the homeless. Some, however, have tested out different skill mixes, for example replacing doctors with nurses, and also different employment relations, for example using salaried general practitioners. A recent review[35] suggested that their impact had so far been limited, but the process they embody – that of planned piloting of ideas for service development – is an important one, to which we will return in later chapters.

The design of care for specific needs

The National Health Service serves a wide range of needs, but for most of its life there was not, for each need or group of needs, an accepted process for determining how they should best be met. Professional bodies have made a large number of proposals aimed at improving service delivery but, though such contributions have been critical to the development of some services, particularly emergency care, they have not amounted to a comprehensive or systematic process for designing how care is delivered.

Such a process began to take shape in the 1990s.[36] As we have noted, the London Implementation Group reviews identified serious weaknesses in the structure of London's hospital services, and in respect of cancer that concern became national. *The New NHS* proposals for national service frameworks were presented as a follow-up to the approach already adopted for cancer services.[37]

In fact, the original report was very broad brush and fell far short in specifying exactly how services should be delivered and what was needed to improve performance. As a subsequent review[38] pointed out, the proposals failed to take into account a wide range of factors, particularly the staffing implications of the proposals. Moreover, the report contained no information on the costs of the proposals or the scale of the expected returns in terms of lives saved and lives extended. In several respects, therefore, it fell short of being a service plan. Nevertheless, this report and the national service frameworks that followed established the principle that services should be consciously designed.

At local level, the development of care pathways represented the emergence of the same principle, albeit on a smaller scale. Gradually, the term came to be used in official documents to describe any attempt to relate services to users. In 1998, the NHS Executive advice for the definition of long-term service agreements – the replacement for contracts under the old regime[39] – stated that the agreements '... will engage all those who contribute to a pathway of care' (annex C). It adds that this approach means the agreements will have to be developed at the level of the service rather than the institution, and will '... be increasingly based on Integrated Care Pathways focusing on conditions or client groups rather than organisations' (p 3).

The advice did not specify how this was to be done and since its publication no further guidance has been issued in England[40] on this specific issue. The growing adoption of this approach, though not yet formally evaluated, amounts to a significant improvement and is central to the analytic framework we develop below. As the next section indicates, however, it represents a partial rather than a systematic approach to service design.

The whole system

The term 'whole systems' came into use in official documents around 1997 in a number of contexts, including winter pressures, elective care targets and mental health. Although the National Beds Inquiry focused on hospitals as a whole, much of its analysis bore on services for elderly people, which the report identified as the main users of hospital beds, and on the need for considering the 'whole system', i.e. both community and hospital services, to meet the needs of elderly people.

In the context of winter pressures, the need for a whole system approach became apparent as the NHS responded to repeated crises during the winter period. From the mid-1990s, hospitals were struggling to cope with the pressure of demand for emergency medical admissions during the winter months. Peaks of demand, whether in the early winter caused by flu or other chest complaints or around the New Year, led to hospitals closing their doors or stacking up patients on trolleys in corridors.

The Centre was slow to react, but in 1997 a task-force identified a large range of measures to relieve the pressures on hospitals that involved working across traditional boundaries and which recognised:

- that the crisis in a hospital might, in part at least, be resolved by action outside it
- that the independent responses of the various providers might not produce the best overall response.

In the case of elective care, the Government came to power committed to reducing the numbers recorded as waiting for elective hospital care. In its view, that required an increase in elective activity. It had to recognise, however, that there were other claims on hospital capacity, particularly from emergency patients. Accordingly, in 1998 it issued a circular[41] setting out a range of measures that might achieve a better balance between the different demands being placed on the hospital, principally the competing claims of elective and emergency patients.

In neither this nor subsequent circulars, however, is the term 'whole system' very precisely defined. What precisely is 'whole' and what is meant by a 'system'? No official document set out the underlying logic but the term, nevertheless, rapidly came into general use.[42]

In practice, as these instances of its use indicate, the 'whole system' is not the whole system, i.e. the whole of the NHS, still less the environment within which it functions. But in all these cases its use embodies some of the key features of the definitions cited in the foreword, particularly the interaction between different services and different elements of a particular service. Explicit recognition of these represents a significant step forward, one that will be developed in the following chapters.

The structure of the workforce

Many aspects of the UK NHS reflect specific policy interventions by the government of the day, such as the 1962 Hospital Plan that led to the creation of a network of district general hospitals. But in large measure the structure of the system as it now stands is not the direct result of policy from the Centre but rather from developments within the workforce that have been driven by external forces, principally the growth of clinical knowledge. These, to the extent that they have been controlled, have been under the direction of professional bodies rather than government. This is particularly true of three of its central features:

- the hospital–community divide
- specialisation within the hospital
- professional roles across the Service as a whole.

The divide

The central structural feature of the NHS is the division between hospitals, where medical specialists work, and the community, where generalists work. As Honigsbaum[43] has shown, the hospital–community divide, already apparent in Dawson's time, was confirmed by the establishment of the NHS, i.e. by the deal that Bevan struck with the medical profession. Although this division has been questioned from time to time, in general it has remained an apparent constant in the system, with only minor deviations occurring. In some small hospitals, for example, GPs retain admitting rights to beds but in total these represent only a minor part of the bed stock.[44]

Although the 'divide' remains a fundamental feature of the NHS, a great deal of effort has gone into a range of measures designed to bridge it by creating effective working links between hospital and community-based clinicians. The notion of shared care, for example, emerged during the 1980/1990s,[45] while the total purchasing pilots[46] led to a number of projects designed to alter the boundary of work between community and hospital, such as outpatient consultations within general practice.

But, while these measures appear to have been beneficial,[47] they have largely been the result of local initiative and remain limited in scope, in both geographical and professional terms, and in respect of the conditions they cover. However, the development of national service frameworks also bears on the links between hospital and community-based services, covering as they do all the clinical interventions bearing on a particular condition. So far, these have been prepared within the existing division of roles between hospital and community. As we shall see later, some developments point the way towards change in the way that these roles are defined, but that challenge has yet to be posed in a fundamental way.

Specialisation

A second fundamental feature of the NHS, which it shares with all other advanced health care systems, is clinical specialisation, particularly among the hospital medical workforce. This structure has largely developed of its own – the apparently natural consequence of the growth of clinical knowledge – and therefore a *sine qua non* of higher standards of care. Despite its importance to the way that services are delivered, the question 'specialisation in what?' has generally been treated as not needing an answer in public discussion.

Throughout the inquiries of the Royal Commission on Medical Education[48] and investigations by the Social Services Committee (as it then was) of the House of Commons into medical training,[49] the issue was not raised.

While there has been some concern about the extent of sub-specialisation, the larger picture has mostly gone unchallenged, even though from time to time voices have been raised against it. In 1980, for example, a report from the Medical Manpower Steering Group[50] expressed concern about the development of further specialisation within the medical profession, fearing it would make it over-rigid and unable to respond to changes the Group could not foresee in the workforce the Service would need in future.

Many of the pressures that have led to the existing level of specialisation are still present. Professional support for larger hospital units[51] continues to be based on the belief that greater specialisation will offer better care. The process of developing national service frameworks has led to more rather than less emphasis on specialisation in the whole of the clinical workforce.

Not everyone has automatically viewed such development as desirable. For example, a 1996 report entitled *The Future NHS Workforce*[52] raised a series of objections to current developments, while its successor report[53] put forward fundamental proposals for changes in training and career development. These, however, fell short of attempting to define what the appropriate basis and extent of medical (and other professional) specialisation should be, taking the NHS as a whole. As we shall see below, some professionals have argued that the current pattern of specialisation is inappropriate for some of the care the NHS has to deliver. But the broader question remains to be addressed on a systematic basis.

Professional roles

Essentially the same issues arise between professions. Their present structure can be explained historically, by events in the nineteenth as much as the twentieth century, when the branches of the medical professions emerged – particularly the division between surgeon and physician and between hospital and community practitioners and when the medical profession succeeded in limiting the aspirations of other professions such as midwifery and nursing.[54]

There have been some signs of movement at the edges of many professional interfaces, such as the introduction of nurse prescribing and the devolution of clinical responsibility to nurses for service delivery, e.g. in midwifery. But change has been slow. In 1997, the Audit Commission suggested that the NHS might benefit from following the US in using nurses as anaesthetists,[55] a proposal that had been made decades earlier, but there has been no response so far.

It has long been recognised that service needs should determine how professionals are trained, i.e. which particular bundles of skills they have and which measures should be taken to ensure that those skills remain up to date. But, because the force of history and precedent is so strong, nearly all discussion of the structure and balance of the Service has to start with a set of largely predefined building blocks. *In the Patient's Interest*,[56] a report by the Standing Medical and Nursing & Midwifery Advisory Committees published in 1996, set out a large range of measures designed to support professionals from different disciplines co-operating and co-ordinating across organisational boundaries.

But, proposals such as these took the existing professional boundaries as given. The need to consider more fundamentally the links between workforce and service planning was finally recognised in full by the Health Select Committee report[57] published in 1999, which argued that the existing structures for workforce planning should be radically redesigned. As noted in Chapter One, the government response acknowledged the need for a fundamental review, and a consultation document followed in early 2000. While this did not consider the fundamental determinants of professional roles, it did recognise that, in the past, the Royal Colleges in particular had played a key part in determining how the medical workforce was structured, but these organisations, by their very nature, are built round tight definitions of professional roles. Later in the year, the Government's *NHS Plan*[58] announced a series of changes designed to reduce the impact of professional boundaries. The Plan proposed that:

> *... appropriately qualified nurses, midwives and therapists [shall] undertake a wider range of clinical tasks, including the right to make and receive referrals, admit and discharge patients, order investigations and diagnostic tests, run clinics and prescribe drugs.* (para 9.5)

These proposals represent a major change from the relatively tentative relaxations of professional boundaries that have taken place in the past, often on a local and experimental basis.[59] If the Service responds, then the way is open for the fundamental redesign of specific services based on new job definitions that stem from the needs of the patient rather than the professional.

The role of users

Health care is largely delivered by professionals; it is therefore no surprise that until recently it was the professional view of how services should be provided that dominated. This has begun to change.

The rhetoric of 'users first' became stale with repetition,[60] but it has slowly begun to move towards being a reality, much of the pressure to change coming from patient groups themselves.[61] In the case of maternity care, a report from the House of Commons Social Services Committee[62] concluded that the views of users should be given greater weight in determining how the service should be designed. In the face of professional objections, it argued that women should be given the choice between hospital and home, and should be allowed to accept the risks that choice might involve. That recommendation was subsequently take up by the Government in *Changing Childbirth*, and a slow process of changing the pattern of service delivery was begun.

At a more general level, in 1997 the Conservative Government launched *Patient Partnership*, which recognised that patients were and could be in a position to decide what form their treatment should take.[63] Subsequently, in its White Paper, *Saving Lives*, the Labour Government took the further step of acknowledging that patients might be experts in their own conditions.[64]

These developments in part reflect general trends in society, from deference to assertiveness. Within health care itself, two other factors have been particularly important: the rise in the importance of chronic conditions, due in large part to increases in life expectancy; and the increasing availability of clinical knowledge in electronic and other forms. As a result, some patients are in a position to determine themselves what form of treatment they need, albeit often with the advice of a professional.

The NHS Plan took the further step of describing the Government's vision for the NHS as 'a health service designed around the patient'. It went on to set out a series of proposals in line with this vision, including specific services such as rapid response teams and general criteria such as speed, convenience and high quality. In these ways, the user perspective is at last being given greater weight, but the further step of designing the whole structure of the NHS around the user has yet to be taken.

Conclusion

The NHS at the end of the twentieth century would still have been recognisable to Dawson. The GP gatekeeper role has scarcely changed and in some ways been strengthened through the transfer of purchasing power of hospital services first to fundholders and then to primary care groups. The sharp division between the role of the community-based and the hospital-based professional also remains. In the hospital sector, the division between the local district general hospital and the larger teaching hospitals also persists, albeit in a less extreme form. Within primary care, general practice continues to be small scale, with a large number of practitioners remaining, as had been the case at the turn of the century, single-handers.

Furthermore, the rhetoric of *The New NHS*, by virtue of its repetitive emphasis on working together, underlined the failure of the NHS to do so. In other words, despite the developments recorded above, what was seen as a fundamental weakness decades before has not been resolved despite, as Box 2.1 indicates, a vast amount of rhetoric devoted to doing so.

Box 2.1 Terminological profusion

Integration	Working together
Joint planning	Whole systems
Joint working	Inter-professional/disciplinary working
Co-operation	Teamwork
Collaboration	Shared care
Building bridges	Joined-up government
Partnership	

But a great deal has changed. The financial and organisational framework within which each part of the Service worked is radically different. More important is the shift of emphasis from organisations and administrative processes to service delivery itself. The policies introduced by the new government recognised:

- the need for an explicit process of service design based on broad need groups such as cancer sufferers or specific functions such as intensive care for children
- that for some tasks the system, i.e. all service providers rather than the individual service, has to be addressed
- that staffing and service issues should be considered jointly and the workforce should be defined in terms of the work that needs to be done rather than traditional professional roles
- that services, not institutions, are the proper focus for designing the delivery of care.

- that the emphasis in planning care for broad need groups such as cancer sufferers should shift from specific interventions to the context in which they are applied
- that services should be designed around the individual user, not the professional

But while these developments, once they emerged, seemed self-evidently valuable, they have yet to be brought together into a coherent whole and their implications fully thought through. Despite the emergence of 'whole systems' in official documents, in practice both policy and implementation have been partial, typically confined to a particular service or institution. The NHS Plan, for example, is built up from a series of apparently independent initiatives that, even when added together, do not represent a comprehensive treatment of the full range of services the NHS delivers.[5]

Furthermore, the bulk of the effort devoted to the improvement of care during the 1990s has been devoted to episodes of care. Within the NHS, the drive for clinical effectiveness, and outside it the development of the Cochrane collaborations, have largely focused on the clinical- and cost-effectiveness of specific procedures or of measures to deal with specific problems.

In the UK and elsewhere, the vast majority of the resources devoted to enhancing the knowledge base of health care delivery has been on specific interventions – new drugs, new means of diagnosis and new forms of surgical procedure.[6] It was not until 1991 that the NHS began to develop an explicit policy towards R&D in relation to its services, but the programmes launched as a result remained largely focused on clinical topics such as cancer care. However, it did include elements such as the primary–secondary interface and the policy research programme that examined parts of the wider context in which clinical interventions took place. But it was only in 2000 that the Service Delivery and Organisation programme was launched, focusing specifically on the way that care is organised and delivered. Consequently, as later chapters will bring out, very few of the issues with which this book is concerned have attracted substantial attention from researchers.

So, although the elements for a systematic approach to the delivery of health care services were beginning to emerge in the late 1990s, they still had to contend with both institutions and frames of mind that were inimical to it and a knowledge base that contributed little. Research and policy continued to be commissioned and developed in separate compartments, and training and service delivery were still largely determined by separate forces.

Thus, by 2000, the NHS had still to find a way of integrating policy-making over the full range of issues considered in this chapter. Although the new government had launched a wide range of initiatives bearing on key aspects of the overall structure of the NHS, it had not explicitly attempted to make effective links between them. As the King's Fund noted in its response to the report of the National Beds Inquiry, there was a need to:

> *Bring together all the relevant strands of policy, including national service frameworks (particularly those for Older People and for Mental Health), the private finance initiative and the capital planning process in general, workforce planning, including the current review as well as the funding and organisation of long term care. At the moment, these interconnections are not being made. The capital investment strategy ... published last year – signally fails to do this and the workforce planning consultation document ... does not give systematic attention to the likely trends in service delivery nor to the particular problems identified here. The private finance initiative remains focused on the individual trust rather than the local health economy.* (p 6)[67]

Such an integration of policy across so many areas is an extraordinarily difficult task given the wide range of considerations that come into play. Whether such an agenda can be tackled effectively will be considered later. Before doing so, we turn next to developing the ideas or conceptual framework that underlie the improvements identified above.

References

1. Guillebaud, 1956.
2. In spite of this conclusion, the Committee felt it was premature in their view to reorganise the Service at that early stage of its development.
3. Subsequent Green and White Papers (Ministry of Health, 1968, 1970, 1972) came to similar conclusions.
4. Royal Commission on the NHS, 1979.
5. Fundholders received budgets to be used for the purchase of (most of) the elective care their patients required.
6. The use of contracts to integrate services is supported in King's Fund Management College, 1996.
7. NHS Management Executive, 1991a.
8. Mays *et al.*, 1998.
9. See Audit Commission, 1997a, or Clinical Standards Advisory Group, 1998b, for examples of such failure.

10. Secretary of State for Health, 1997.
11. Prior to this, the merging of the main funding streams was possible only within the framework of the 1997 NHS Act.
12. Dawson, 1920.
13. The health centre is a concept whose time is always about to come.
14. Ministry of Health, 1962.
15. Department of Health and Social Security, 1980b.
16. Department of Health, 2000g.
17. Department of Health and Social Security, 1986.
18. Secretary of State for Health, 1986.
19. The Department of Health paper on the role of trusts (1989) contains no reference to this issue.
20. Tomlinson, 1992.
21. Department of Health, 1995.
22. See National Association of Health Authorities and Trusts, 1993.
23. However, changes in medical training also made it difficult for smaller hospitals to continue to provide the full range of acute care.
24. London Implementation Group, 1993.
25. Standing Medical Advisory Committee, 1997.
26. Scottish Office, 1998.
27. This term is also used by Monaghan *et al.*, 1999.
28. NHS Wales, 2000.
29. Malcolm, 1991, 1994.
30. Taylor, 1989.
31. See National Association of Health Authorities and Trusts, 1994.
32. Secretary of State for Health, 2000.
33. Department of Health, 2000g.
34. Department of Health, 1996, 1997.
35. Jenkins, 1999.
36. The early 1990s saw the rise of evidence-based medicine. But, with a few exceptions, this was and remains focused on the evaluation of individual interventions rather than the full range of interventions serving a broadly defined need or need group.
37. Department of Health and Welsh Office, 1995.
38. Cancer Research Campaign, 1997.
39. Department of Health, 1998a.
40. See, however, Welsh Assembly, 2000.
41. Department of Health, 1998.
42. The mental health national service framework, for example, refers to the whole systems approach as though its meaning did not require any explanation.
43. Honigsbaum, 1979.
44. Although the division appears fundamental to the NHS, there were those who, in the early days of the NHS, considered that it had been a mistake that would eventually have to be reversed, primarily because it undermined continuity of care.
45. See, for example, Edwards *et al.*, 1996, and Hickman *et al.*, 1994.

46. Mays *et al.*, 1998.
47. Levy, 1997.
48. Royal Commission on Medical Education, 1968.
49. House of Commons Social Services Committee, 1981.
50. Medical Manpower Steering Group, 1980.
51. See, for example, British Medical Association, Royal College of Physicians of London and Royal College of Surgeons of England, 1998.
52. Health Service Management Unit, 1996.
53. Health Service Management Unit, 1999.
54. Rafferty, 1997, Rafferty *et al.*, 1999.
55. Audit Commission, 1997.
56. Standing Medical and Nursing & Midwifery Advisory Committees, 1996.
57. House of Commons Health Committee, 1999a, 1999b.
58. Secretary of State for Health, 2000.
59. McKee and Black, 1991.
60. See, for example, Department of Health and Social Security, 1979.
61. Mackenzie, 1979.
62. House of Commons Health Committee, 1992.
63. Cumberlege, 1993.
64. Department of Health, 1999b.
65. It contains, for example, no substantive discussion of emergency care or community health services.
66. This is discussed in Harrison and Dixon, 2000, Chapter 12.
67. In autumn 2000, however, the Secretary of State announced that, in future, hospital schemes would have to be considered within the context of the local health economy.

PART TWO

Analytic framework

Chapter Three

From pathways to systems of care

Chapter One began with a thought experiment: what would the ideal health care system look like? The previous chapter recorded how, in the real world, attempts have been made to modify the structure of the NHS so as to answer that question, albeit never in a sustained and systematic way. Instead, change has been piecemeal and much of it unplanned and unanticipated by the Centre.

But that criticism is easier to make than to respond to. For what emerges from Chapter Two is the complexity of the task, once all the elements of it are considered together. If all the fundamentals – the scope of formal organisation, the design of services, the definition of professional roles – are called into question, where is the firm ground on which an attempt to find the answer can be based?

If, as the rhetoric has it, 'services are for patients', then it must be found with users and their perceived need for care. The first part of this chapter, therefore, takes the individual patient journey and sets that in the broader context of a 'system of care' or group of pathways. The second considers the arguments for using pathways and systems of care as the basic building blocks for the design of health care delivery. At the end of this chapter, we comment briefly on a more traditional approach that uses the concept of primary, secondary and tertiary levels of care as the key to system design.

From pathways to systems of care

As a first step towards developing an alternative approach, we begin with the notion of a care pathway – the series of events that occurs, or the states users must pass through in the search to obtain care and, where they are successful, return to their starting point.

For most patients, most of the time, the care pathway is very simple – it consists of a single visit to a GP or other professional to resolve a particular problem. A key element in the case for a locally provided service such as general practice, and the other disciplines often to be found in conjunction with it, is the fact that most care episodes involving professionals are of that type. A health care system consisting only of such simple pathways would pose few design issues and the pathways themselves present few difficulties for their users.

But for some patients the care pathway is complex and lengthy. It may consist of a long series of encounters with different professionals in different organisations. At various points along the way, the route may fork and offer choices of different treatments in different locations. At any point, the patient may 'opt out' and decide not to continue further, or to seek care outside the formal, professionally based care system through either self-help or the services of complementary therapists such as aromatherapists.[1]

The typical complex and extended care pathway is fractured, its signposts are unclear, and there are no mileposts to indicate the user's rate of progress along it. As Bruster *et al.*[2] found in a study of hospital patients:

> *Before they arrive at hospital, patients often receive no information about the hospital. When admitted to hospital they may be told little about their daily routine. During their stay in hospital they are often not informed about their condition or treatment or about tests and operations, and they are given little opportunity to discuss these matters with staff … At discharge patients are rarely given information about how they should continue with their lives when they reach home.* (p 1545)

What patients engaged in a long care journey actually want is the reverse – a clear route through the health care system and clear signs along it: in principle, that is what the care pathway offers. In the words of a proponent: [3]

> *The Pathway acts like a map for the patient, letting them know where they are going, what they are likely to come across on their journey, and when their journey through the particular episode is likely to end. In this way, the patient is better informed, and thus more able to participate in their own care.* (p 9)

From the patient's viewpoint, a well-designed pathway is clearly part of a 'good' health care delivery system. But a properly designed pathway does more than provide better information to patients: it can also determine the 'best' way of providing the care episodes along the way and the 'best' sequence of those episodes.

As far as we are aware, no one has attempted to define a whole health care delivery system in terms of pathways. Nearly all attempts to define pathways have been 'bottom up', led by practitioners in the field[4] wishing to reform the part of the health care delivery system they work in or know best. Precisely because they have been developed from the ground up, there is no standard terminology (see Box 3.1 below) or definition of what exactly the determination of a care pathway involves. But it may involve any or all of the following:

- definition and adoption of best clinical practice drawing on all the available evidence
- elimination of duplication, e.g. of tests or requests for information from patients
- redesign of the sequence of care
- better communication between professionals
- changes in professional roles
- continuous monitoring of performance.

Both the patient experience and the way that care is provided can be radically altered by the formal definition of a care pathway, and both clinical and economic benefits may ensue.[5,6]

Box 3.1 Terminological profusion yet again

Integrated care pathways	Patient-focused care
Multidisciplinary care pathways	Clinical integration
Critical care pathways	Integrated service networks
Anticipated recovery paths	Organised delivery systems
Disease management	Collaborative care programmes

In practice, the changes following the introduction of a care pathway are limited in scope. Most formally derived pathways are confined to a single institution or even one function within it, and to a single often quite narrowly defined category of patient, such as someone being treated for a hip fracture. Hence, the implementation of a care pathway usually involves a 'slice' of the work of a particular institution, typically a hospital.[7] There are practical examples of where pathways have been defined across institutional boundaries from the start to the end of a care episode, but these are relatively few.

In some cases, however, the emphasis *is* on the links between providers – on all the elements of the care system that contribute to the treatment of a particular condition. The notion of disease management, for example, is based precisely on this consideration (see Box 3.2) This takes, typically, a chronic condition such as asthma and aims to ensure – through measures bearing directly on professional roles, such as treatment protocols, and indirectly, such as contracts running across organisations combining their contribution – that the best combination of interventions is provided for patients.

Box 3.2 What is disease management?

- a knowledge base that quantifies the economic structure of a disease and includes guidelines covering the care to be provided, by whom, and in what setting for each part of the process
- a care delivery system without traditional boundaries between medical specialties and institutions
- a continuous improvement process that develops and refines the knowledge base, guidelines and delivery system.[8]

That 'best combination' comprises what we term here a *programme of care*. The national service frameworks for coronary heart disease and mental health are programmes of care in this sense. They define for each patient group the type of interventions that should be offered, the range and standard of facilities and the number and type of professionals that should be available They cover all the providers involved from the initial contact through to the final end-point of successful treatment and recovery.

National service frameworks have, up to now, been developed for a small number of conditions. Disease management programmes have also been developed for only a limited range of conditions largely of a chronic nature, such as asthma. Neither has been developed by taking the whole health care delivery system, breaking it down and developing programmes or frameworks for each part.

The next chapter considers how the whole system of health care delivery might be divided up into programmes of care. Before considering that question, we first develop the ideas underlying both care pathways and disease management. While pathways and programmes of care are critical elements in describing how health care delivery does and should work, neither goes far enough. Although both focus on particular groups of patients, they rarely attempt to include the behaviour of patients or of professionals. In other words, they do not embody those characteristics that, following the definitions set out in the Introduction, characterise systems: interaction between the various elements of which they consist.[9]

At the level of the individual pathway, the focus is (almost) always on a pre-existing and known number of patients flowing along it. Similarly, but with less justification, the initial attempts to define national service frameworks for specific user groups also ignore the nature of the interaction between patient and the health care delivery system.

To bring out the significance of this omission, we set out in Box 3.3 the various ways in which the UK NHS offers a response to a perceived need for urgent care.

Box 3.3 Urgent care response in the UK

Hospital A&E department	Pharmacy
Minor injuries unit	Walk-in centre
GP surgery	Ambulance
Out-of-hours co-operative	NHS Direct

The key features are:

- there are many entry points
- users decide where and when to enter
- the same functions are carried out by different providers, e.g. minor problems may be dealt with in at least three different settings and all may offer advice as well as treatment
- there is a choice as to where some functions are carried out, e.g. telephone advice may be provided at any of the sites involved or completely separately
- patients may be passed between providers, e.g. the GP may call an ambulance and send a patient to the A&E department
- there are several routes back to home or other end location, some direct and some via intermediate facilities such as nursing homes.

Figure 3.1 overleaf shows that the NHS response to users' requirements for urgent care consists of a number of pathways, some of which intersect. These present a set of options from which, as things currently stand,[10] users are free to choose the most appropriate, in the light of their own assessment and perception of their needs, and the most convenient personally. In what follows

Figure 3.1 A whole system view of emergency care

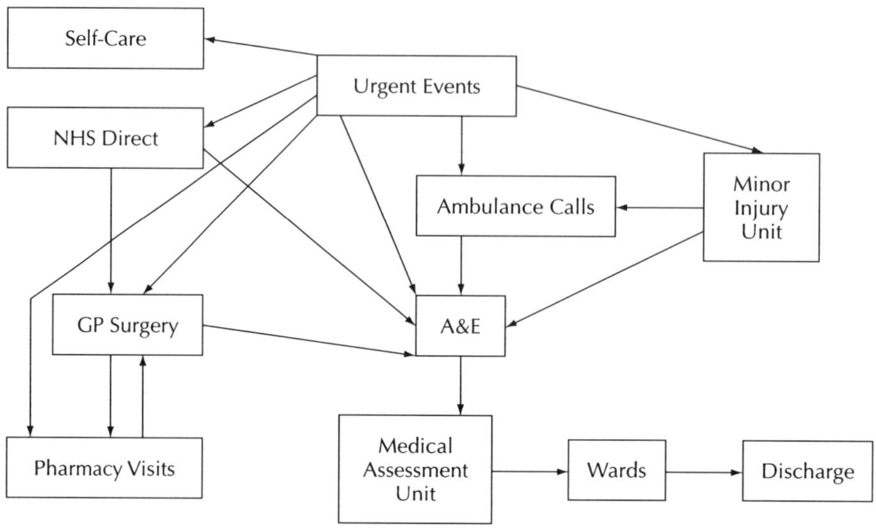

we use the term *system of care* to refer not only to a set of closely related pathways but also to their users and the way they interact with those pathways.

In the case of urgent care, the case for considering all the pathways set out in the diagram together as one system is obvious enough. Although the services involved treat conditions ranging from the trivial to the life threatening, they combine to meet a fundamental requirement from the user point of view – the need for an urgent response to a perceived need for treatment. It may not be apparent at the outset what the nature of the response should be. A condition that the user considers trivial may turn out to be life threatening, and vice versa. Thus, a central task for the professionals working in different parts of the system of urgent care is to determine just what speed of response is appropriate when the patient presents with what he or she perceives as a problem, and hence in which part of the system it should be dealt with.

In making these decisions, professionals may also be influenced by their expectations or knowledge of the state of other parts of the care system in which they work. They will, of course, be influenced by their professional assessment of the patient's condition, but other factors may also come into play, including an assessment of the nature of the options that are available and the time it may take to access them.

In contrast to the simple pathway, therefore, knowledge and information pass around the system of care in a number of ways and those participating in it respond in their different ways. Some of these responses may be codified in terms of agreed protocols or decision rules. In practice, most reflect unwritten and often unarticulated custom and practice as well as the assessment of the professional decision-makers of the likelihood of certain elements of the pathway being promptly available. For example, decisions on whether or not to refer a patient to a hospital A&E department may depend on the GP's assessment of the likelihood of the patient being seen quickly or the time it will take to get there.

As a result of both user and professional decision-making, the numbers flowing through the system vary according to system performance (the delays or other features it presents to individuals) and to its configuration (how close the facilities are to where people live). Thus, system design and system performance influence the level of use that the care system experiences both in total and in its constituent elements.

In contrast to urgent care, access to non-urgent elective care within the NHS is largely controlled initially by the GP and then subsequently by the hospital specialist. Nevertheless, it too can be described as a system of care.

In outline terms, the elective care system can be seen as a simple pathway, as in Figure 3.2.

Figure 3.2 The pathway to care

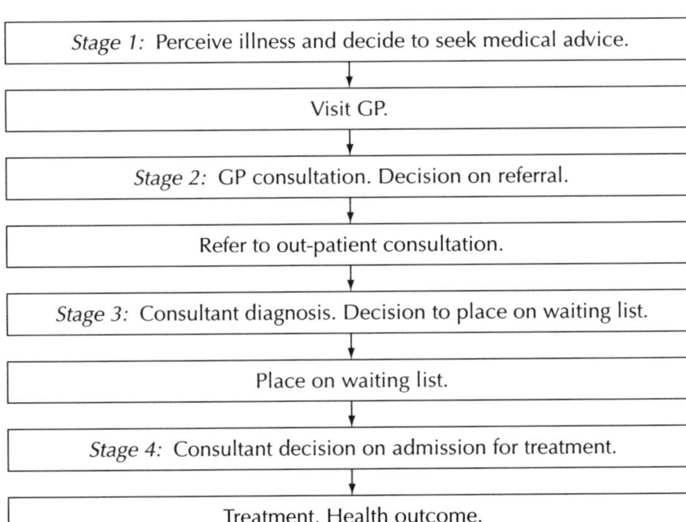

Despite the apparent simplicity of the pathway shown in the figure, the case for considering elective care as a *system* is underpinned by exactly the same considerations as apply to urgent care. At any point on this simple pathway, a decision may be made to leave, in the light of both personal and professional expectations of what moving to the next stage involves. Figure 3.3 illustrates these choices.

Although the figure does not show this explicitly, each stage represents a decision on the part of the user whether or not to proceed further along the pathway. That decision will, of course, be in part determined by the nature of the professional advice received, but it may also be influenced by other factors including the availability of other options and the expected time it may take to reach the next stage. The advice offered by professionals may, as with urgent care, depend on their assessment of how easy or difficult it may be to gain access to the next stage of the pathway.

While these interactions are widely recognised, they are also widely ignored. As we have argued elsewhere,[11] policy towards elective care has been based on the premise that demand for care does not respond to access times, and as a result

Figure 3.3 The elective care system

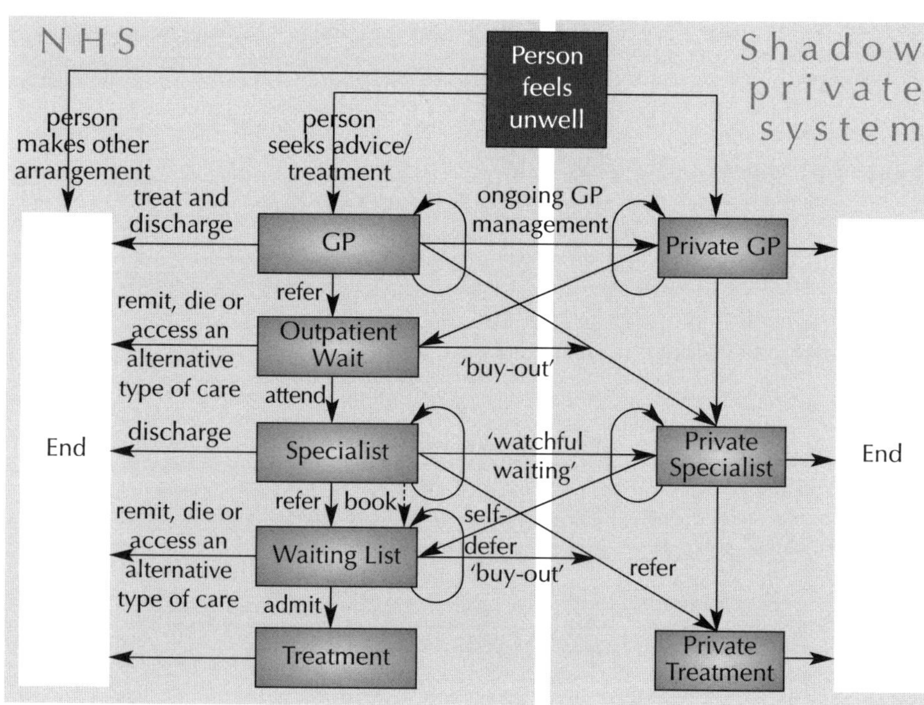

Source: Hamblin *et al.*, undated.

targets have been set for reducing numbers waiting that have persistently been missed – precisely because more users came forward when waits fell (and for other reasons as well). The evidence suggests that both users and their professional advisers (generally GPs) respond to what they know or perceive of the system 'downstream'. Similarly, the key decision-makers further along the pathway – the hospital consultants – may also be influenced by the numbers of patients coming forward and the availability of beds and other facilities required for treatment.

The system of care set out in Figures 3.2 and 3.3 can be seen as representing the pathway faced by one individual. It can also be seen as the first step towards defining the care pathway for a particular procedure or as a representation of a wider national system, i.e. all the patients who seek and receive elective care in a particular locality or the country as a whole.

In the latter case, the pathways may not be linked at all and may not represent alternatives to the individual user: the pathway for cataracts, for example, will be quite distinct from that for joint replacement. The case for considering them together rests on the assumption that, though they are distinct, they work under similar rules and similar pressures. In other words, it is a useful analytic convention to treat them as one system of care. It has practical significance as well, because at national level targets have been set both for the reduction in the total number waiting for elective care and for the maximum time people should spend waiting.

The elective and emergency systems of care set out above represent virtually the whole of the health care delivery system. Each is founded on the central

Box 3.4 Definitions

Care pathway: a single 'map' of the way in which a single category of user gains access to successive episodes of care and defines the nature of that care at every stage.

Programme of care: a set of closely related pathways, e.g. for a disease like cancer.

System of care: this embodies the first two but allows, in addition, for behavioural interactions between users and professionals and between each of these and the system of care itself.

Whole system: all the services or other components that are involved in health care delivery within a national health service. It therefore comprises all the above, for all users.

notion of the pathway and of the patient seeking care and of proceeding along a pathway to obtain it. Scale apart, the key differences between a care pathway and a system of care are:

- the system of care consists of a (large) number of interrelated pathways
- the patient's decision to enter the system may be made in the light of the current state of the system (i.e. whether it is busy or not) as well as its general characteristics (i.e. whether it is convenient to access or not)
- people may leave if the system does not respond to what they want or not quickly enough
- professional behaviour is influenced by what happens or is assumed to happen in other parts of the system
- each part has its own rules or constitution, stemming from their different organisational forms. Thus, the way that financial and other resource constraints work within hospitals differs from they way they work on GPs.

This last point is not inherent; as we shall see, it is possible to imagine a care system that operates under consistent rules which all those within it respect – what we will term a *managed system of care*. As things currently stand within the NHS, however, there are no large systems of care managed or even partially managed in this sense. Thus, while access to specialist care is controlled by GPs, how they do that is almost entirely discretionary. The same is true of the way that hospital specialists decide whether or not a user, having been referred by the GP, proceeds further along the pathway. Furthermore, professionals typically do not see themselves as part of a wider system of care: instead they remain largely focused on their own element of it.

Gradually the introduction of national service frameworks and clinical pathways will change that. But as things currently stand, the notion of a system of care remains largely an analytic one. The next section considers the arguments that might be used to justify using it as the basis for defining, in practice, how the health care delivery system as a whole should be structured.

Why systems of care?

Figures 3.1, 3.2 and 3.3 have some interest in their own right as descriptions of how the NHS works, even more so when they are allied with data showing the numbers of people going down each of the paths. Using local and national data (Figures 3.4 and 3.5), we can shed some light on the relative importance of the different providers to users.

Figure 3.4 A local care system: who uses what?

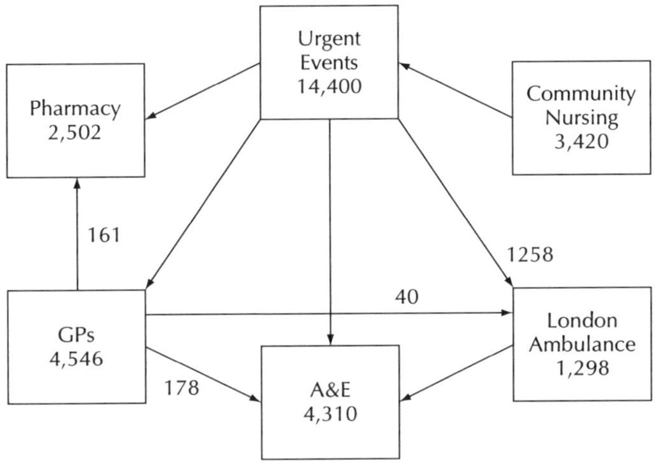

Source: Boyle *et al.*, 1998.
Note: the survey on which this figure is based was carried out over a Bank Holiday weekend in Lambeth, Southwark and Lewisham in 1998. At that time, NHS Direct was not available

Figure 3.5 Access to elective care 1996–97

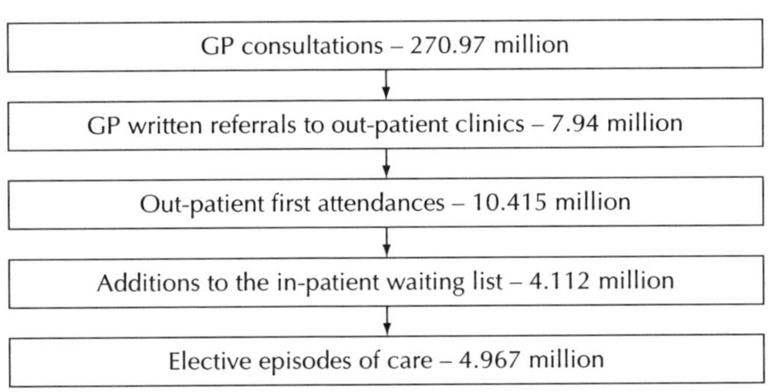

Source: Harrison and New, 2000.

In Figure 3.4, it may come as a surprise that as many people use a pharmacy as go to their GP. It may be a surprise of a different sort that in general the figures set out above cannot be supported by data on the numbers flowing through the system of care. The data used in Figure 3.4 resulted from a special survey carried out in three London boroughs. The data shown in Figure 3.5 for the elective care system derive from national sources at a very high level of aggregation. Using these allows only the outline of each system to be illustrated.

These gaps reflect the fact that the NHS – like other health care delivery systems – does not routinely collect data on a system of care or pathway basis. Nearly all the data collected nationally refer to specific providers: the same is true of nearly all the data collected locally, including clinical audit data. We return to this point and some exceptions to it below.

Even where data are not available, however, figures like those shown above may be a first step towards understanding how far a care system extends and which range of providers has to be taken into account to grasp how it works. The figures themselves, however, shed only very limited light on the strength and the nature of the connections between providers. But, as the definitions cited in the Foreword suggest, it is the interconnections and the resulting interdependence that underpin the case for using the care system as the basic unit of analysis, as we now go on to show.

Functions not institutions; or who should do what

The definition of a care pathway for a small patient group requires the specification of clinical roles and routing or transfer rules, as well as the definition of the appropriate intervention at each stage of the pathway. As noted above, implementation of a care pathway can change who does what, how it is done, and, less commonly, where it is done. Essentially the same applies to systems of care for broader groups of patients.

Within any care system, we can identify a number of distinct roles played by professionals, each of which may in turn divided up into further elements:

- advice
- diagnosis
- care
- routing/sorting patients to the appropriate place for diagnosis and/or care
- communication (and transport)

There are two key notions involved in determining which agency or profession carries out each of these, or any element of them. The first is *unbundling*, i.e. taking the elements of what a provider does and considering whether all currently need to be carried out in the place or by the same organisation, and the second is *substitution*, i.e. one provider taking over a task from another. These two processes go hand in hand.

The critical point of a focus on function rather than institutions is that to do so detaches what is done from the provider agencies and the professionals that currently do it, and allows new options involving different divisions of roles between agencies or professionals to be identified.

In the case of the hospital A&E department, it has been generally assumed that if a patient can be treated there, he or she should be. But recent developments such as pre-admission wards are based on the perception that the key task of the A&E department is determining *what* should be done: the decision as to *who* should do it is a separate issue. This perception[12] leads not only to pre-admission wards, where more time and information is obtained about the state of a patient before the decision to admit is made, but also to defining links with community services and a redesign of how they work so as to allow patients to be returned tocommunity settings where clinically appropriate.[13] In this case, the unbundling of diagnosis/decision/treatment allows new pathways to emerge that may be cheaper and/or more effective for some patients than admission to hospital, which was at one stage the only option if further treatment or care was required.

NHS Direct provides another example of unbundling. Before its introduction, some GPs and some A&E departments offered telephone advice,[14] i.e. the advice was linked closely to existing providers. NHS Direct has unbundled the advice from the provision, opening the way for a comprehensive advice service that functions independently of any care, diagnosis or transport provider.

The unbundling process is critical to examining both the professional role and the functions of specific organisations. As the citation from the SMAC report indicated (page 20), changes within hospitals have undermined their self-sufficiency and required decisions as to which aspects of a programme of care for a specific client group are carried out where – and the 'where' may be hospital or community. The development of systems of care provides the opportunity for the existing bundles – professional and organisational roles – to be examined and re-assessed away from their existing institutional context.

Financial and other spillovers

What one part of the health care system does may affect the costs or the workload of others. Essentially, there are two ways of dealing with these interactions or spillovers: to bring them all within the same organisational and financial framework (i.e. to *internalise* them); or to provide means of compensating for them, through financial or other mechanisms.

The case for disease management has been based on the first of these. Its proponents argue, for example, that higher drug costs on one part of the pathway reduce costs further along it. Unless the system of care – in this case one based on a particular disease – is provided within a 'whole care system' financial framework, the provider responsible for the higher drug costs may be unwilling to incur them. Without such a framework, the incentives facing each provider discourage the most efficient method of provision.

More typical, perhaps, is the reverse situation, where the way that one provider acts puts up the costs to others (or reduces the chances of a successful outcome for the patient). The classic example is over-rapid discharge from hospital, which leads to community-based providers having to give extra support to compensate for the shorter stay, possibly at greater cost than an extra day in hospital.

This phenomenon may also be internalised through merger of hospital or community services. The alternative is to use the system of care as an analytic device to define the best division of roles between hospital and community and then to devise financial arrangements which as far as possible guarantee that it is in the interests of the providers involved to deliver care in line with the 'best division', e.g. by creating a budget covering all post-operative care, held jointly by hospital and community or by an independent purchaser.

Incrementalism is not enough

The search for the 'best division of roles' is not, however, sufficient to define the best overall way of delivering a system of care. The typical way in which health care delivery is improved is for one provider, or group of professionals within that provider, to modify the way that it provides its contribution to a care system. But, while most improvement in health care delivery takes place in this way, it does not necessarily lead to the best overall system of care. A key insight obtained from taking a broader view is that each provider may provide the best possible care and yet the system of care as a whole is not the 'best possible'.

In the example just given of over-rapid discharge, the apparent need is to improve the capacity of the hospital itself. But taking a system-wide view may suggest that the way to improvement could lie in measures that may bear on the inflow of patients and hence reduce admissions. Alternatively, the appropriate response may be the development of services within the community that can deal with more dependent patients.

More significantly, the system-wide view may lead to identification of gaps in current provision that an incremental approach would not reveal. In the case of care for the elderly – which, as we suggest later, can be seen as a care system in its own right – the UK pattern of provision appears to have neglected the potential for rehabilitation after discharge from acute care.[15] Incremental improvement in the way hospitals or general practice operated did not lead to the development of this function.

In part, this gap reflects the effects of policies designed to pursue other goals. In the last 20 to 30 years, many community hospitals to which patients transferred after a period of acute care in a larger hospital have been closed. But the scope they offered for intermediate care may be precisely what is required in the interests of the overall care system.

There is a close link here with financial spillovers as again the issue is one of incentives. In the case of intermediate care, as UK experience has shown, there may have been no provider with the financial incentive to provide it. Its benefits may accrue to both hospital and community providers such as GPs. But as each has its own financial responsibilities, it is not sufficiently in the interests of either one to ensure it is available.

Within the examples given above, another key notion can be identified, that of *feedback*. The acute hospital may, in the interests of its own drive to cut costs, shorten lengths of stay and reduce turnover intervals through 'hot bedding', which allows hospitals to work at more than 100 per cent of nominal capacity. But that may impose costs on community-based services that have to provide aftercare for patients who are not yet fully recovered. They may in turn cut back measures such as preventive or anticipatory care, which may lead in turn to an increased hospital workload. In trying to improve its situation, the hospital has only made matters worse for itself.

Feedback can, however, work beneficially in a virtuous rather than a vicious circle. In this example, a virtuous circle may be set up if extra community services are introduced that reduce the need for hospital care and which in turn allow the hospital to provide a more rapid response to those patients who remain, which in turn leads to a reduced need for community services.[16]

Put in this simple and direct way, the point is obvious. In practice, the difficulty is that feedbacks of this kind may be slow to show themselves. Indeed, they may never be observed because they are masked by other changes that are going on within the health care delivery system as a whole. And, as noted already, the nature of the data systems that are currently available means they cannot be identified without special investigation.

Targeting interventions

We take this in two stages, first by considering the patient's progress along a care pathway and second by considering the design of the pathway itself.

Within a care pathway, e.g. for cancer care, the patient may pass through a series of stages where delays may occur. If delay is important, then taking the system as a whole helps to identify where delays are occurring throughout the care pathway and where they can be most efficiently reduced.

This may seem trivial, but for most of the life of the NHS policies designed to reduce delay in access to hospital have been focused on the queue for treatment, not the waits that occur before that stage, either within the community or in the hospital while the diagnosis is being established.[17] Not surprisingly, therefore, the number of studies that map the delays occurring along the whole pathway is very small. Some very obvious conclusions may emerge from studies of this type. In the case of cancer, for example, a study[18] carried out in a US hospital found very long delays at the diagnostic stage. Another study[19] in a British hospital also found long delays at this stage, in this case because of poor organisation (presumably) within the relevant parts of the hospital. More importantly, it identified long delays for some women patients between symptom identification and first contact with the Service. *Prima facie*, both these areas appear to be worth targeting ahead of delays at other stages in the care pathway.[20]

The issue is also a matter of cost and finding the best affordable set of interventions to improve a specific pathway. Programmes of care such as the NHS Cancer Plan and the national service frameworks simply set out what is essentially a clinical shopping list of services, staff and equipment. Once cost or other constraints such as a shortage of skilled personnel in particular categories enter into consideration, choice has to be made from the shopping list.

In principle, setting out all the elements of a system of care enables such choices to be made more effectively. In practice, that may be difficult, not simply because each item on the shopping list has not been fully evaluated in its own right, but also because their interactions have not been allowed for. The NHS Cancer Plan and the national service frameworks implicitly assume that the benefits from the various components they embody are simply additive. But they may not be. In the case of cancer, for example, both patient education and formal screening programmes are designed to encourage early presentation. How much effort it is worth devoting to the latter depends in part on the effectiveness of the former.[21]

Managing demand and utilisation

A key function of the health care delivery system as a whole is to ensure that demands on it are kept in line with resources available. This task is carried out within the NHS in a variety of (largely implicit) ways. But as the example of elective care shows, that function may be undermined by the way that individuals respond to any service improvement. If improvements in access lead to more users entering the system than it can cope with, then some other means of controlling access, such as clinically defined thresholds that determine when a patient should proceed along a pathway, may have to be used.

Similarly, as suggested in the previous section, demand on the various elements of the urgent care system may be interconnected – that is, each is to some extent a substitute for the other. The increase in emergency attendances at hospital may in part be attributable to changes in the availability of community-based services, particularly for those seeking to access it at short notice or out-of-hours. Because of these interconnections, demand management is a system level function: change in the way it is carried out in one part will impact on another part.

On a day-to-day basis, providers have no control over the number and nature of those claims. All health care systems must, therefore, have a capacity to deal with variations in demand.[22] In the UK, this capacity lies largely with the hospital, but that capacity has been overstretched in recent years. The focus in the hospital has been on its own performance, particularly the rate at which day surgery was introduced, not the care system as a whole. Hence, pursuit of efficiency within the hospital has led to a reduction in the overall capacity of the system to deal with variation.[23] The successive attempts to plan for 'winter pressures' can be seen as a search to find the best way, taking the system as a whole, of meeting uncontrollable demand.[24]

To sum up: we have set out in this section a set of arguments for using the system of care as a fundamental unit of analysis of health care delivery. Before developing this approach further, we briefly consider an alternative approach, based on the notion of hierarchy.

Why care systems are to be preferred to hierarchies

As noted above, an early attempt to define an ideal health care delivery system was made by Lord Dawson and this colleagues in the 1920s. A recent critique[25] of the American and British health care delivery systems contrasted the Dawson approach with that in the US to the latter's detriment, and argued that:

> *One concept is essential to understanding the topography of any health care system: the organisation of care into primary, secondary and tertiary levels.* (p 160)

The authors of this critique regarded this division as a universal and desirable feature of health care systems. They then contrasted the ordered approach of the UK to the less structured and more fluid approach of the US and then set out a number of common criticisms of the way that the US has implemented the three-level approach.

As the authors indicated, this way of describing health care delivery systems can be found in the Dawson report,[26] which, as noted in Chapter One, set out a model system of health care delivery consisting of primary and secondary health centres. The report set this out in an abstract figure and then imposed it on a real place – Gloucester and its surrounding area.

The hierarchy of primary/secondary/tertiary rests on an assumed division of roles between the various tiers. But, as Dawson recognised, changes in the cost and availability of medical technologies means that roles are not static. In his day, appendectomy in the hospital had replaced treatment at home with poultices and drugs. Since then, many other treatments have moved into and out of the hospital, sometimes more than once (e.g. stomach ulcer treatments).

It follows that the issue is not the balance between primary and secondary care, but rather whether services were better delivered in one location, i.e. a hospital, or in many, i.e. a general practice or local health centre. This is a matter of the relevant technology and its economics – if the price of MRI scanners fell as fast as computing costs every surgery would have one – and of the importance of the links between functions.

As we have shown elsewhere,[27] the hospital is glued together by the need for physical contiguity for some of its functions. But the glue is not equally strong for all activities. From the early 1990s onwards, research, experiment and practical experience showed that for a range of functions hospital and community are close, indeed often very finely balanced, competitors.[28] Furthermore, as we shall see below, some functions can take place in hospitals but be controlled by community-based professions, i.e. a shift in control may take place, without any shift in location.

Similarly, the distinction between secondary and tertiary rests not so much with a progression from one to the other as with whether or not all services can be provided in local hospitals. The reasons why many cannot be provided in a local hospital, as opposed to regional or national centres, stem primarily from clinical specialisation and its presumed link with quality of care as well as other functions such as training and research.

As Chapter Two made clear, however, the UK version of the hierarchy model does not guarantee that, in practice, health care delivery will be properly structured nor that its component parts will have the right relationship to each other. More fundamentally, it does not guarantee that patients reach the right part of the health care system relative to their needs, even if the majority do.[29]

Evidence of this kind might be countered by the pragmatic argument that unless a health care system has a structure of the appropriate hierarchical kind, it cannot be effective in cost or clinical terms. It is, in other words, a necessary but not a sufficient condition. In practice, many of the policy initiatives cited above reflect this view.

The argument developed here runs rather differently. It accepts, as did Dawson, that different functions within a health care delivery system have different economic and clinical characteristics and hence will tend to be housed in different locations and that some will commonly be found and some rarely. But, as the allocation of activities between locations reflects changes in technology and other factors, the question of whether an activity is secondary or primary is beside the point. The content of the work of the general practitioner is not to be found by the search for the essence of 'primary' activity but rather by considering what, with modern technology, a person trained in that way can do working outside the hospital, either individually or supported by the range of co-workers comprising the community-based care team.

Use of the hierarchy model reinforces the persistent tendency to identify particular service functions, e.g. the provision of first contact care with particular organisations and a particular label – primary care. In fact, there is no clear and commonly accepted definition of primary care. In the UK, it is often used to include a range of services that are quite distinct from general practice, e.g. community pharmacies. Some other European countries, even those that work in a similar way to the NHS, are not identical to it in their range of provision nor in respect of the rules governing the role of the community-based doctor.[30]

Furthermore, hierarchy implies a flow upwards, leaving open the question of the return journey. But for many the return journey is problematic, i.e. it does not simply involve a move back to home but rather the beginning of a complicated road to recovery. Many patients require successive elements of community-based care and so the way that community-based services are organised is as critical to their effective care as the way that hospital-based services are organised.

As the evidence briefly referred to above indicates, the 'return journey' has been persistently neglected and badly organised precisely because it has not fallen clearly to any one 'level' to plan for it. The provision of stepdown or intermediate care including rehabilitation has, in the UK and elsewhere, fallen between the interests of the hospital and the interests of the community-based physician. Instead, it has typically been left to nurses and indeed voluntary bodies to press the case for including these institutions in the spectrum of care.[31]

The final charge to be made against the hierarchy approach is that the hierarchy is the wrong 'metaphor' or mental model for thinking about health care delivery. Although the use of the term 'hierarchy' within health care does not have the connotation of control, it does have that of the superiority of the 'higher' levels. That implication has no relevance to the services actually provided. If we take a particular function, such as the provision of emergency care, the role of the hospital A&E department overlaps with that of a number of other services including general practice, pharmacy and community nurses. All are front-line, point of first access services.

To sum up: persistent though the primary, secondary and tertiary (even quaternary) terminology is, it is a poor way of describing how a health care system actually works or how it should work. It has remained attractive because it has embodied some key features – control of access to secondary care and a broad-based community service – which many regard as crucial structural features of a 'good' health care delivery system. But once those are in place, it has little further value.[32,33]

Conclusion

We have argued that the concept of a system of care, consisting of a series of closely related pathways, is a more illuminating way of thinking about health care delivery systems than a hierarchical division into 'levels' of care. Focus on pathways and still more on systems of care have the central merit of focusing away from the individual clinical decision to the broader context in which that decision is taken, and hence to the various sources of interdependence between different elements of the overall system of care. It also has the merit of taking attention away from specific formal organisations and labels such as hospital or primary care, and focuses it on the functions or tasks to be performed. Finally, it emphasises the patient journey, which should of course be the centrepiece of any system of care.

If the structure of health care systems can be seen as a series of care systems, a series of questions follow:

- how many care systems should there be?
- how and where do they interact?
- how are they combined within an overall system?

These questions form the subject of the next chapter.

References

1. Aromatherapists may, of course, come in from the cold, as osteopaths did, and enter the scope of the NHS.
2. Bruster *et al.*, 1994.
3. Johnson, 1997.
4. Johnson, 1997.
5. These benefits have not been rigorously demonstrated. Ellis and Johnson, 1997, note that ' ... no scientific research has been completed in the UK that evaluates properly the impact of using pathways'. However, they add that '... the growing evidence cannot be ignored'.
6. See de Luc, 2000, for a discussion of different approaches to pathway development that emphasise different elements of this list.
7. Monaghan *et al.*, 1999, make the same point (para 3.34) about so-called 'whole systems', i.e. that despite the use of the word whole, the focus remains firmly on the part.

8. Hunter and Fairfield, 1997.
9. We have used the word 'interaction' rather than 'linkage' to bring out the potential for different elements of a care pathway to influence the way the others work, rather than the simple fact of connection.
10. We consider below some suggested modification to the existing access routes. A report prepared for the Department of Health on out-of-hours services (Department of Health, 2000i) also proposed changes to them.
11. See Harrison and New, 2000.
12. This is inherent in the atrium approach, attributed to Muir Gray, to the role of the A&E department, which sees the department as neutral ground between hospital and community.
13. One example is the nurse-led rapid response team, which can be used at short notice to support someone at home if hospital admission is not needed but some degree of care and observation is required.
14. Crouch and Dale, 1998.
15. Audit Commission, 2000b.
16. This example is considered further below.
17. The NHS Plan does not appear to fully recognise this as the time targets it sets for access to elective care do not explicitly include the diagnostic stage.
18. Billings and Wells, 1996.
19. David, 1997.
20. This point may seem too obvious to be worth making. The lack of evidence on where waits occur suggests it is worth emphasising. Furthermore, even though the present Government has, in the NHS Plan, acknowledged that it is waits that matter, not numbers waiting, the Plan itself falls short of committing the Government to achieving maximum waits taking into account the whole care pathway. The existing targets do not, for example, allow for the time patients must wait after their first outpatient appointment.
21. Mulligan, 2000b.
22. In the case of extreme emergencies, the UK NHS has special standing orders that require the suspension of the 'normal' pattern of activity.
23. The government response, through the work on winter pressures, has been to introduce a whole systems approach. But this approach has not asked the fundamental question of where the capacity to deal with variation can be most effectively provided and where the most effective measures to deal with variation may be found.
24. See, for example, Department of Health, 2000k.
25. Grumbach and Bodenheimer, 1995.
26. Dawson, 1920. See also Fox, 1986, pp 56–7, who describes the development of BMA policy towards hospital provision as working within a hierarchical framework.
27. Harrison and Prentice, 1996. Within all health care systems, professionals generate demands on other parts, on behalf of their patients. The same issues therefore arise with them: they too may add to demands if they see spare capacity emerging. For

example, if in a system of cardiac care more capacity is added to carry out major surgery, it is likely that more patients will be directed towards it, particularly if other treatment modes appear tightly constrained. Again, clinical thresholds or other criteria have to be brought in to manage demand, usually through informal decision-making at local level. We consider these below.

28. Fulop *et al.*, 1997.
29. The evidence for this can be found in nearly any report from the Clinical Standards Advisory Group and the Audit Commission.
30. See Semple-Piggott *et al.*, 1997, for a comparison of The Netherlands, Denmark and the UK, and Gervas *et al.*, 1994, for a more wide ranging comparison.
31 Even in the UK, with its well developed system of general practice, some have argued that the implicit message in 'hierarchy' is pernicious – that it implies a status ranking. As a result, too much emphasis on the top tier (the specialist element housed in prestigious and expensive physical establishments) at the expense of the lowest (the general element housed in simpler premises, if at all). For this reason they want to see it inverted with the patient, or primary care at the top.
32. Shortell *et al.*, 1995, argue that the hospital hierarchy must be replaced by a heterarchy and that the hospital should become relatively invisible '... hidden within the context of more integrated health systems operating as part of community care networks' (p 154). Their integrated health systems are our systems of care.
33. Perhaps the main reason why the hierarchy concept maintains its hold is that the split between primary and secondary coincides with the role of the GP within the UK NHS as a gatekeeper to specialist care and some other hospital facilities, e.g. diagnostics. But for a range of other services, patients can access what they require by a number of different routes. In some cases, specifically dental and optical services, patients do not go through the GP gatekeeper. Nor do they for some hospital services. In two important areas – mental health and emergency care – the standard progression does not work. In both cases, patients can and do present themselves directly to parts of the care delivery system other than their general practitioner for their 'first contact' and in both cases other clinicians have critical gatekeeping roles.

Chapter Four

From systems of care to overall structure

We have argued in the previous chapter that patient journeys should be the analytic building blocks for describing health care delivery, that these should be grouped into systems of care, and that the overall national system should be seen as consisting of a series of systems of care, with each system comprising a number of pathways.

If we accept that systems of care are the right 'unit of analysis', a series of questions arises:

- on what basis should each system of care be defined?
- how many should there be?
- how far should they extend?
- how do they all fit together?

Defining systems of care

The previous chapter illustrated only two systems of care, elective or non-urgent, and urgent. But while these two, with their emphasis on the critical importance of time to gaining access to treatment, are widely recognised ways of describing the elements of a health care system, there is a number of other criteria that might be used for dividing a national health care system into systems of care.[1] These criteria are set out in Table 4.1.

Disease management has typically focused on the first of these criteria, taking chronic conditions such as asthma as the basis for defining a system of care: so too have the first national service frameworks, which have focused on mental illness and coronary heart disease. But a framework has now been produced using the third type of criterion – the user group, in this case elderly people. Elderly people are major users of the coronary heart disease system of care as well as others, such as cancer care, diabetic care and so on.

While the criteria may overlap,[2] they may also be used in combination. For example, the combination of disease and type of patient may lead to a separate

Box 4.1 Systems of care: alternative bases

- disease – cancer, stroke
- part of the body – ophthalmology, ENT
- patient type – maternity, paediatrics, geriatrics, schoolchild, worker, armed services
- treatment mode – radiology, surgery
- function – intensive care, general practice
- degree of urgency – emergency, elective: acute/episodic, chronic
- provider type – hospital, community

system of care such as cancer care for children or old age psychiatry. Others may conflict: for example, if urgent care is taken as a system in its own right, then it may comprise elements of all the disease-based systems. Whether these latter are organised and managed as part of one urgent care system or whether urgent care needs are dealt with within each disease-based system is a central question for the overall design of a health care delivery system.[3]

Yet other 'labels', such as radiology or intensive care, are commonly used for parts of health care systems. Although these make sense because they are attached to a well-understood function, they cannot form systems of care in their own right since they represent only part of any care pathway. Rather, as argued further below, they are best described as services that contribute to systems of care.

The same is true of that most familiar of labels, the hospital. Although it is common to refer to the 'hospital system', the hospital itself is not a system of care. The hospital, within the present framework, embodies a wide range of elements, some of which belong to most systems of care, and some of which belong to only one. It is not a system of care as we have defined it.

Different countries use the criteria set out in Box 4.1 in different ways to produce different service structures, but as far as we are aware no country has attempted to establish its overall health care delivery system according to a set of consistent principles. Furthermore, the professional literature generally does not do so either. Instead, each profession or part of each profession has attempted to stake out the ground that it can occupy, using whatever criteria best suit that purpose.

At this stage in the argument we too do not want to set out a 'right' answer. Instead, we withhold judgement as to which of the criteria should, in isolation or in concert, be used as the basis for defining systems of care, precisely because it is where the criteria conflict that the most important structural issues arise and where debates about the structure of health care systems are most intense.

A simple health care delivery system

Within a health care system such as the NHS, with a well-developed network of general practice, the existing specialty structure in the hospital defines, for the general practitioner referring patients to hospital or to community-based specialties such as mental health, the 'boxes' to which they route or to which patients route themselves where the system rules allow them to do so. The result is shown in very simple form in Figure 4.1.

The GP making a referral decision has to determine which of the 'boxes' created by specialisation is likely to be most appropriate – in effect, which system of care the patient belongs to. This task can be described as routing or sorting patients into the appropriate box. Within this simple model, the GP is part of all systems of care by virtue of being the main gatekeepers to all of them.

Essentially, Figure 4.1 represents a series of vertical divisions of the hierarchy model. Had this diagram been drawn up 40 years ago, it would have looked very different. The number of 'boxes' would have been much smaller and hence the task of the GP much simpler. With obvious exceptions, such as maternity, there were essentially two main options: general medicine and general surgery.

Figure 4.1 A simple structure: GP as router

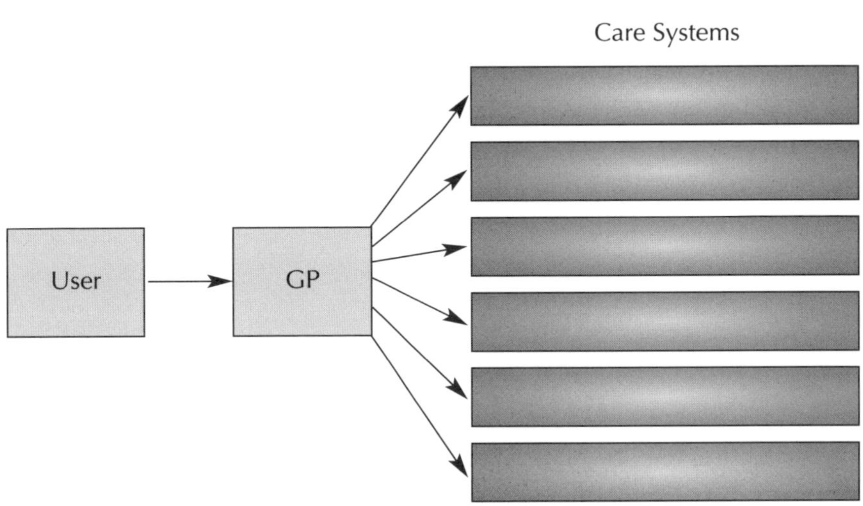

Now there are 30 to 40, depending on the precise complement of each hospital – more if the further sub-specialties are counted in the total.

This identification of specialties with actual or potential systems of care begs the question of whether the divisions that have arisen within the roles of hospital-based physicians and surgeons are the right basis for defining systems of care. As we shall see in more detail below, the structure of specialisation has largely been created by professional pressures rather than as a considered response to the range and types of needs the health care delivery system has to deal with. But for the time being we will assume that the specialty divisions represent the starting point for determining boundaries between care systems.

Interdependence between systems of care

In principle it would be possible to imagine a national health care delivery system consisting of a series of independent care systems. In other words, once a decision had been made as to how to divide up the national system into systems of care, each might then be organised according to its own particular characteristics – the number of its clientele, the personnel and equipment it needs, the degree of specialisation, and so on. As McKeown argued[4] when he proposed his age-related split, the aim should be to find relatively homogeneous groupings: ideally, they should also be chosen so as to minimise the links between them, i.e. they should be more or less self-contained.

In some cases, such groupings can be identified. Some community health services, partly for historical reasons and partly because some of the clinical links between these and other parts of the health care delivery system are relatively weak, are provided outside the NHS itself. For example, community eye services, now almost entirely provided by the private sector, are largely independent of the rest of the NHS in organisational, financial and physical terms. Community opticians may identify conditions such as glaucoma or retina detachment that they cannot treat and which they therefore recommend patients to have treated elsewhere. But for the most part their work is self-contained. The same is true of dentistry. In both cases, there are hospital-based services as well but the links between these and community-based services are relatively infrequent. For most patients, most of the time, opticians and dentists are effectively independent, an independence underlined by their private contractor status.[5]

In earlier decades, other parts of the NHS were also substantially separate – some hospitals were devoted purely to maternity care while community midwives, and to a lesser extent health visitors, were devoted almost exclusively to the care of mother and child. However, hospital policy since the Second World War has been designed to bring together what were once physically separate systems of care.

Over the years, the UK has drastically reduced the number of hospitals devoted to specific conditions such as infectious diseases (because their importance has diminished) or hospital-based maternity care (because of the presumed risks of isolated units). They have not altered the broad pathways, except in a geographical sense, along which patients must travel. But, as a result, what were once independent systems, or system elements, have become parts of a larger set of interdependent systems, particularly within the hospital, where these once physically distinct services now call on facilities used by other systems of care.

Within hospitals, pathways and systems of care come together in space, i.e within one building, because:

- they share expensive diagnostic equipment and other facilities
- clinicians contribute to more than one pathway
- clinicians perform other functions in the hospital, such as teaching or research
- the pathway the patient should be on is not always clear, so patients must be brought together within, for example, the A&E department or admission ward to be routed on to the appropriate pathway. The hospital, like the GP, has a routing or sorting role.

In the hospital, the work of each consultant (and team) connects through the use of the same theatres or diagnostic facilities, support facilities and so on. Some connections matter only part of the time, e.g. when investment in new capacity is being planned, or where the siting and availability of support services is being considered, or where changes have to be made to the share of these facilities each enjoys. Other connections, particularly those that bear on the contribution of some specialists to the emergency care hospitals provide, are continuous and critical to the way each care system operates.

The extent of this interdependence is increased by the way in which UK hospitals provide emergency care. Within the UK hospital system, many if not the majority of hospital physicians and surgeons are part of both the elective and the emergency care system as, except in the largest hospitals, they take part in a 'take' rota for the admission of emergency cases. This double role is, as we shall see, an area of continuing difficulty.

The same issues arise outside hospitals. Systems of care outside hospitals, such as those for mental health, are less dependent on physical facilities. But they nevertheless require the orchestration of professionals with different skills who belong to more than one system of care. In the case of mental health care for the young, as an Audit Commission study[6] has noted, many professionals work in more than one system:

> *Psychologists and speech therapists, in particular, have a wider remit than mental health, and are often core members of other teams that deal with disability and physical health However, having their own separate caseloads and referral routes puts another obstacle in the way of co-ordinated child and adolescent mental health services.* (p 63)

As suggested in the previous chapters, a system (or programme) of care can be seen as comprising elements from a series of contributing services. In some cases these elements lie entirely within the same care system, i.e. A&E within the emergency care system, but in many others services contribute to several systems of care.

In what follows we use the term 'service' to refer to a professionally defined element of the health care delivery system rather than one defined by patient needs: services and systems of care may coincide but in many if not most instances they do not. Thus, as noted above, services such as radiology form only part of any care pathway, but they contribute to many such pathways, which in turn will form part of different systems of care. In contrast, a service such as that provided by emergency ambulances falls (almost) entirely within the emergency care system.

The linkages between *services* and *systems of care* are the main source of the complexity of health care delivery systems. They make it impossible to define the boundaries of a system of care with any precision. Even if we use very broad definitions, such as the emergency–elective divide used in Chapter Three, there are important linkages between them. They intersect where they use resources in common. Hence, for some issues, the 'whole system' must mean exactly what it says – the whole of the health care delivery system.

Extending care systems into the community

The simple health care delivery system set out in Figure 4.1 rests on a sharp division of role between the GP and the specialist. That division is often regarded as a fundamental and beneficial feature of the UK system. In this section we consider its compatibility with the development of systems of care.

In the simple system set out in Figure 4.1, the prime role of the GP is that of router. Nevertheless, the hospital remains the locus of a great deal of sorting or re-sorting activity. The need for this is greater in the A&E or emergency side of the hospital since many patients present themselves while others have been referred by GPs because of uncertainty about the appropriate diagnosis. In addition, hospital specialists cross-refer to colleagues in the light of diagnostic or other investigations. The scale of this re-sorting activity reflects a number of factors: the ability of the GP to select the right box, inherent clinical uncertainty as to the nature of the patient's condition and multiple morbidity, which means that patients might require services from several 'boxes'.

While the growth of clinical knowledge has led to the growth of hospital – and some community – specialties, it has also altered the nature of the routing role. Through open access schemes, community-based physicians are now able to draw on diagnostic facilities (albeit they remain sited in the hospital) and in this way they increase their ability to determine which 'box' or system of care each patient is best sent to. In effect, the routing role has in part been transferred from hospital to community.

The same considerations arise at the point of hospital discharge. Again, there may be a series of options, and hence a routing decision has to be made as to the appropriate next stage in the patient's journey, be it returning home or progressing to an intermediate care institution or to terminal care. The patient journey may continue further in terms of time, if it requires the contribution of the wide range of professionals working in the community. The basic requirement, to ensure that these contributions are properly related in time and place, remains the same as in the hospital. Who should carry out this role – the GP or the hospital – is less clear, but the role itself goes beyond routing, to the 'orchestration' of the different elements required by a specific user.[7]

The GP is also a care giver. Community medical care could be said to be a system in its own right for all those conditions that do not need the resources of the hospital. But if systems are defined on the basis of disease or user characteristics such as age, then the GP in the NHS (though not, as we have noted, in other countries) contributes to all of them.[8] In the national service framework proposals for coronary heart disease and mental health, GPs appear as contributors alongside a range of other professionals in hospitals and the community.

While this is a fair representation of the current situation, the growth of clinical knowledge that led to specialisation within hospitals is to a lesser degree also present in the community. This raises the question of whether GPs can continue to be a part of all health care systems, particularly if they develop, as foreshadowed in the national service frameworks, towards being managed systems operating under defined rules.

As long ago as the 1960s, McKeown argued[9] that general practice in its then form could not be sustained. His proposals not only combined specialisation by age groups but also the extension of the (specialised) GP's responsibility to hospital care except for certain specialist areas, where the then existing and still current system of referral would continue. In his words:

> ... *a more satisfactory basis for the future of medical practice would be provided by basing domiciliary care on four types of doctors – obstetrician, paediatrician, adult physician and geriatric physician – working in groups whose composition would be determined largely by the age of the related population. Each would function as a personal doctor and would be responsible for hospital as well as home care*. (p 178)

As this extract indicates, McKeown's case rested in part on the value of continuity to the patient but also on the implications of the growth of clinical knowledge for the general practitioner role. In his view, this growth meant that it was impossible for any one clinician to cover the span of work that general practice comprises. Others have taken a similar line.

In 1976, a committee chaired by Professor Court[10] recommended the introduction of general practitioner paediatricians on similar grounds. Some children's services developed out of local authority provision and entered the NHS in 1974 as organisationally distinct, with the result that the NHS contained two parallel systems, one based on clinical medical officers and one on GPs.

The committee's central aim was to bring together all preventive and curative health services bearing on children within one integrated child health service – to establish, in other words, a system of care for children, staffed by properly qualified people. To this end, the committee proposed that some GPs should be more thoroughly trained in paediatrics and work as general practitioner paediatricians, concentrating on, but not solely dealing with, children.

These proposals aroused strong hostility from the medical profession, despite their modest nature, on the ground that it would undermine the concept of a *family* health service. Court emphasised that he did not envisage a break-up of the general practitioner system but it appeared that way to his critics, and the notion never took hold. A system of care for children has still to be developed, running across all providers of care to children.[11]

The same arguments have been applied to other services. A recent report[12] – the first national survey of GPs involvement in mental health – proposed both more training in mental health issues and some degree of specialisation, either within large practices or between the practices making up a primary care group. As the report notes, this already occurs to some degree both in mental health and in other areas, through the process of informal intra-practice referral.[13] The MACA report notes that:

> *There seems to be at least the possibility for some form of win-win arrangement, whereby GPs wanting to do more mental health work take on a specialist role, whilst those wishing to do less compensate by taking on additional non-mental health consultations.* (p 6)

The case for specialisation of this kind stems in part from the aim of 'shifting care to the community'. This slogan has a clear meaning for those groups such as the mentally ill and the learning disabled who were once cared for in large institutions. The implications of their care being moved to other locations is that the specialised professionals who provided it in long-stay hospitals have to be recreated within the community setting. In these cases, a whole care system has moved physical location and its content changed. This process may overstretch general practice.

As the report pointed out:

> *This [specialisation] may be difficult for small and single handed practices, and it is only likely to work with larger practices, groupings of practices or even PCG wide collaborative working. This will be much harder than it sounds and*

a high degree of creative thinking will be required. However, if a cross-PCG approach to specialisation can be achieved, it will be the beginnings of corporateness, upon which the success of PCGs depends. (p 6)

The logic is the same, if less clear cut, for the community parts of other systems. In the case of cancer, the NHS Cancer Plan proposes[14] that there should be lead clinicians based in the community. It does not suggest that they should become points of first contact for cancer patients, but that would be a natural development at least for some cancers once diagnosis and a treatment plan have been established.

This brief discussion reveals a number of structural dilemmas within the organisation of the 'frontline'. In the simple model, the front-line role is invested in one person, who treats, routes and manages the full range of presenting patients. Those not requiring routing onwards to hospital professionals are treated within the 'general medical system', primarily by medical personnel but also by nurse practitioners carrying out tasks once classified as medical.

At the other end of the scale, the front-line role is disaggregated into areas of specialisation mirroring, at least in part, the hospital, and the treating, routing and managing roles are divided between different professionals. This latter model has been generally resisted in the UK, but as we have noted in relation to cancer and mental health, the pressure to move in its direction seems set to grow, while in respect of eye and dental services users already make the routing decisions for themselves.

From the standpoint we have adopted, the critical question is: which end of the spectrum do users wish to be? The answer may be both: some of the pressures for disaggregation of the frontline into different elements stem from users themselves, particularly those with chronic conditions where the scope for a large degree of self-management is large. At the same time, other users continue to value some of the elements of the aggregated model, particularly continuity with the same professional.

Thus, designing the overall health care delivery system round 'the user' begs the question of whether or not all users want the same thing, or whether any one user wants different things according to the nature of his or her condition. We return to this issue in Chapter Six.

How many systems? The geographical dimension

The extent of clinical specialisation and the geographical scope of a system of care are closely related phenomena. Put simply, the greater the degree of specialisation, the smaller the number of care systems within any given geographical area. Developments over the past century illustrate the point.

In Lord Dawson's model, the care system comprised the city of Gloucester and its surrounding towns and villages and the nearby teaching hospital. Nowadays, that would appear too narrow a geographical definition. The scale of many of the hospital activities has now exceeded the market represented by a relatively small English city.

The Dawson model, like the 1962 Hospital Plan, assumed that with a few exceptions such areas could be self-sufficient. Since the 1960s, the scale at which areas can be self-sufficient has risen, thereby in effect reducing the number of distinct geographical systems from, within England, some 400–500 to some 200. But even this number may be too large for some care systems. The trend towards specialisation has meant that even in a country as large as the UK some care systems are national – and in some smaller countries such as New Zealand (or, closer to the UK, the Channel Islands) depend on the facilities of other countries. As suggested in the previous chapter, it is considerations such as these that underpin the continuing use of the 'layer' or hierarchical model.

Recent developments, particularly in emergency care, have begun to undermine the self-sufficiency of the small town even further. The critical question is the relationship between the emergency role of the hospital, particularly for acutely ill or injured patients, and its other functions. Although hospitals have provided emergency facilities for over a century, the process of developing a properly organised service for this purpose has been protracted.[15] Over the last decade, a series of proposals has emerged, largely from professional bodies, for the provision of such services that would lead to a reduction in the number of hospitals.

In the early 1990s, it was argued that the UK should consist of around 50 care systems, each focused on a major hospital offering the full range of clinical facilities.[16] In effect, this placed the emergency function of the hospital at the centre of the overall care system. More recent proposals have been less radical but have rested essentially on the same presumption. For example, a recent report from the BMA, the Royal College of Physicians and the Royal College of Surgeons argued for further specialisation within surgery,[17] which would mean a major reduction in the number of care systems offering emergency surgery. The logic of this was pursued further in a recent proposal[18] for a national trauma service, i.e. one nationally organised system of care (see Box 4.2).

The key assumption underlying the process of specialisation, as far as the patient is concerned, is that it results in better clinical quality. As we shall see in the following chapter, that assumption can be challenged but, if we accept it for the moment, the critical question in the present context is whether or not other care systems have to match the scale of the largest one. If the answer is yes, and all the hospital-based elements of all care systems would have to move in step, the implication is that hospital facilities should be highly concentrated: if the answer is no, then the implication may be that the existing pattern of hospital provision has to change, in particular, that the notion of a general hospital serving nearly all the needs of a district has be revised. Instead, the role of the local hospital has to be defined in the light of which range of services its catchment area justifies.

Whether all hospital-based services have to move in step depends critically on the nature of the links between the different functions of the hospital. As care is

Box 4.2 A national trauma service

Trauma systems

- In order to improve the care of the severely injured there should be a network of geographical trauma systems covering England, Wales and Northern Ireland.
- Each system would serve a population of up to three million.
- There would be an advantage in a single emergency ambulance service with a medical director for each system.
- The backbone of the National Trauma Service will remain the acute general hospital. In line with the Audit Commission report, there should be a reduction in the number of hospitals that receive major trauma.
- In support of the National Trauma Service, there should be sufficient intensive care facilities for severely injured children, sited in major acute hospitals providing specialist paediatric services. Severely injured children may be transferred to specialist children's hospitals that meet the requirements of a major acute hospital.
- Rehabilitation arrangements for the severely injured must be identified for each system.
- Each trauma system should have an agreed major incident policy.

Source: Royal College of Surgeons and British Orthopaedic Association, 2000.

currently organised in UK hospitals, emergency and other care systems are closely linked and, as a result, the drive to improve or maintain emergency care, which has been assumed to require fewer and better equipped sites, has tended to force others to adapt as well. Developments in paediatrics as well as changes to medical training have had a similar impact. Consequently, the trend over the past few years has been for a reduction in the number of hospitals and a growth in the clientele of each.[19]

But not all care systems or elements of systems are subject to the same pressures.[20] Some elements of most care systems have often remained in the original locations even when other elements have moved elsewhere. For example, diagnostics, outpatient consultations, treatment of minor injuries and day surgery are often to be found in small hospitals that have lost all in-patient functions. In all these cases, the economics of the activity allow 'small-scale' production on site or through the deployment of staff from other sites on a visiting basis. In these ways reasonable access can be retained while not impairing quality of care or incurring significant extra costs.

From the user viewpoint, unpacking from the general hospital those functions that can efficiently and effectively be provided locally is obviously desirable in terms of better access. What the user cannot see, and what is generally unclear even to the researcher, is what is lost or gained by further concentration of those other functions where the professional view supports it. The professional view is rarely justified in quantitative terms, even in respect of clinical outcomes, still less supported by financial or other arguments.[21] Furthermore, it tends to rest on existing methods of provision, including the continuation of existing medical training practices.

Hence, the balance between scale (and presumed quality) and access should be struck remains unresolved.

The whole care delivery system

The term 'whole system' has begun to creep into official documents without being defined precisely. What is clear however is that the 'whole system' rarely *is* the whole system, i.e. all the service elements that a health care delivery system as a whole comprises.

For a narrowly defined group of patients, it may seem a self-evidently reasonable procedure to focus on an individual pathway. For cataract patients, for example, the whole system means all part of the health care delivery system involved in the care pathway. In our terms, this is the system of care for cataract.

Even at this micro-level, however, there are risks that action taken to improve specific pathways or system of care may impose costs in other ways. For example, considered from the viewpoint of an individual pathway through a hospital, a diagnostic facility specific to it will generally appear advantageous, but to 'go independent' may mean that the efficiency of diagnostic services to other pathways is reduced. If there were no costs to this process, this would imply that the hospital as a set of physical facilities did not offer any advantages resulting from joint use. Similarly, the shift to day surgery for this procedure has implications for the ability of the hospital as a whole to cope with fluctuations in demand for beds.

Taking a wider set of services – elective surgical care – the case for isolation of these from the rest of the hospital is clear enough to those working within it. Isolation reduces the risk of operations being cancelled as a result of unanticipated inflows of emergency patients. But such isolation imposes costs on the emergency side by reducing its flexibility at times of peak demand. That spare capacity can be created by expanding the emergency bed stock – but then the combined elective and emergency system may be more expensive as a result. Hence, there is a case for considering 'the hospital system' as a whole. Equally, there may be scope for creating spare capacity in other institutions, e.g. nursing homes. This would involve looking at almost, but not quite, all of the whole delivery system.[22]

It clearly makes no practical sense, however, to propose that any attempt to improve health care delivery within one part of one system of care should always take into account the impacts of any change on 'the whole system'. Judgements have to be made about which interconnections to take into account and which to leave to one side. The following considerations bear on how such judgements may be made in practice.

For analytic and planning purposes, the scope of any system of care extends far beyond the immediate health care delivery system devoted to it. Any consideration of the causes of ill health will expand the notion of the relevant system still wider. Many, if not most, of the policies bearing on ill health lie outside the health care delivery system and outside the clinical domain. Ultimately, this may mean that the system of care, for the purposes of planning and design, includes the global environment. This may seem extreme and impractical but, as understanding of the implications of global warming and the impact of the physical environment on health grow, that perception may alter. Furthermore, unless it is taken into account, the evaluation of the contribution of any care system to the achievement of better health will be impossible.[23]

As the national service frameworks have recognised, a comprehensive programme of care comprises those policies that forestall or anticipate the need for care – prevention, health promotion, surveillance and screening. How these various elements should be brought together, i.e. which organisational, financial or other means should be employed, is considered below. The point here is that any attempt to define a system of care should consider all these, but that does not itself imply that they need to be taken into account on a day-to-day basis.

Any health care system combines other functions – research and training – that have to be reconciled with the provision of care. Unhappily, their economic characteristics are quite different: the requirements of both training and research tend to favour larger institutions (with a full range of patients) than are required for the purposes of service delivery. Furthermore, they fall under different financial and administrative regimes. As a result, these interconnections have been analysed only rarely, even though the development of the hospital system in its present form, particularly the major institutions, can in large part be ascribed to the requirements of these other functions. The balance between them has emerged rather than been determined by a conscious or explicit process.

Again, these interactions need not to be taken into account on a day-to-day basis. But a health care delivery system should embody a process that allows these interests, like competing systems of care, to be properly reconciled.[24] No such arrangement currently exists within the UK. As a result, these separate systems impinge on each other in ill-understood and unpredictable ways.

It follows from these points that 'the whole system' is of massive complexity, the full extent of which has never been grasped in any official review of the shape of health care delivery in the UK. It also follows that the term 'whole system' should be used very selectively. In this text we use it only for health care delivery in its totality. But even this 'whole system' is only part of a much larger one.

While some interconnections need to be recognised only on an occasional basis, others, such as the competing claims for beds and nursing staff of the elective and emergency roles of the hospital, may need to be part of day-to-day as well as long-term planning. The need to explicitly allow for this area of interconnection is now well recognised. Other interconnections, such as those between the development of specialisation and the provision for medical emergencies, have received less attention because their impact is less immediate: we consider these further in the next chapter.

In general, therefore, the question of 'where to draw the line' cannot be answered precisely and once and for all. But, as the examples given above indicate, a key criterion is the timescale of the impact on specific care systems of developments in others. Where timescales are long, impacts can be taken into account on an occasional basis: but where they are short, then either care systems have to be defined so as to include (i.e. internalise) them or means must be created, such as the winter planning mechanisms, to take them into account on a continuing basis.

Conclusion

The move from 'the system of care' to the whole of the health care delivery system has proved far from straightforward. There are different ways of defining systems of care, and choosing between them poses dilemmas, particularly where specific professionals or services contribute to more than one system.

It has proved to be impossible to break down the whole into a series of distinct systems. Instead, interconnections are inevitable and it is these that give rise to the complexity of health care delivery.[25]

The extent and importance of the complexity that the connections between care systems gives rise to underlines again the inadequacy of the hierarchy model as a shorthand description of health care delivery. But it also undermines *any* attempt to divide up the health care delivery system into a set of subsidiary elements.

For this reason, the notion of a Rubik cube may be more a more accurate shorthand description of the whole health care delivery system than a hierarchy or a set of systems of care. The original of Figure 4.2 shown below precedes the invention of the Rubik cube by some decades. The key 'truth' contained in the cube metaphor is that it can be sliced in different ways and that change in any one slice/dimension will affect all the others. This interconnectedness stems directly from the strong links between different care systems and different contributing services.

Figure 4.2 The health care system as Rubik cube

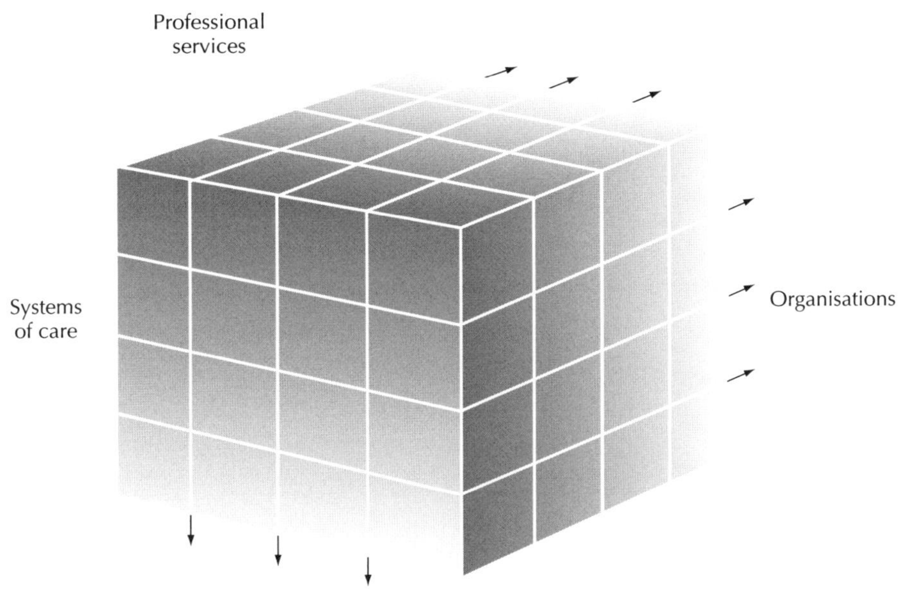

If the various care systems making up a health care delivery system were as tightly coupled together as the Rubik cube metaphor suggests, then the pressure for fewer and fewer geographically determined care systems would continue to produce greater and greater concentrations of clinical resources with no obvious upper limit. But, however great the benefits in terms of particular systems of care, this process would bring with it costs of its own – the costs of access imposed on patients. These set a boundary to the reduction of the number of geographically defined systems, albeit an imprecise one.

Furthermore, the Rubik cube metaphor overstates the tightness of the links between care systems even within one geographical area and hides the extent to which it is possible to counter the pressures for concentration by, for example, unbundling those activities that do not gain from concentration, such as those defined above. Nevertheless, it remains a powerful way of expressing the underlying truth that 'everything connects'.

Another way is the notion of a network (see Figure 4.3 overleaf). The network shows connections in several directions at once: the linkages may represent information flows, patients flows, money flows. Any one element is part of several different care pathways, meeting different needs.

Figure 4.3 Health care delivery as network

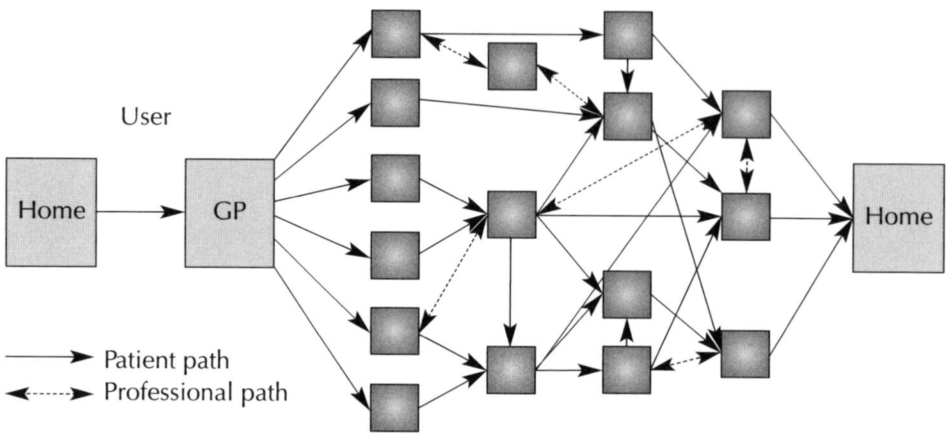

These interconnections stem from a number of different factors, some of which, such as shared diagnostic facilities, are general and likely to occur in all health systems using a similar level of technology, while others are specific to the way that a particular system is organised and the resources available to it. For example, the links between emergency and elective care are not necessarily as close in other countries as they are in the UK, since the way that emergency care in particular is organised differs. In other words, different countries will have different degrees and types of interdependence, reflecting their different clinical traditions and institutions, and their nature will change in any one country in response to clinical, economic and social change.

If everything connects with everything else, then the task of finding the 'best' health care delivery system is formidable. If we take one part and aim to make that 'the best possible', there is a risk that the wider repercussions of such a change will reduce or even negate the hoped-for benefits.

In practice, it is not possible to consider everything at once, but there are no hard and fast rules to determine which parts of the whole delivery system can be considered in isolation or where to find the firm and undisputed ground. The criteria set out in the previous section provide some guides to where 'to draw the line', but in practice it will always be a matter of judgement, made in the light of the decisions to be made at the time.

In other words, in some contexts, such as the strategic planning of health care delivery and the development of policies towards significant functions such as training, the 'whole system' may mean just what it says. In other contexts, it may well be justifiable to draw boundaries around particular areas – systems of care in our terminology – and focus exclusively on them. But there will always be risks in this process.

This conclusion suits the health care analyst who is free to chose 'where to stop'. For other purposes, it not possible to take such a relaxed views: jobs have to be defined, contracts set and organisations built round specific clinical tasks. Such decisions, while not irrevocable, have long-term implications. It follows that if systems of care are to be used to define the structure of a health care delivery system in practice, defining their boundaries and the links between them involves a series of difficult decisions. How difficult will become even more apparent in the chapters that follow.

References

1. There are others. Within surgery alone, 'specialization cleaves surgery along various planes – age, sex, anatomical region, organ system, pathological condition and technology'. Loefler, 1997, p 1.
2. The mental health national service framework does not apply to older people.
3. Some hospitals now have physically distinct entry points for victims of acute myocardial infarction, precisely because of the need to treat that condition very rapidly if it is to be effective.
4. McKeown, 1965.
5. In Lord Dawson's model, however, they would have at least shared premises with other community-based services. They rarely do this now. The vast majority of hospital services, however, are delivered on shared sites, precisely because of the importance of their interdependence. The NHS Plan has rediscovered the virtues of Lord Dawsons's proposals for health centres or, as they are now called, one-stop shops.
6. Audit Commission, 1999b.
7. See Bull, 2000, and Grumbach *et al.*, 1999.
8. The only systems of care lying outside the GP's range are those based on special groups, such as the armed forces or prisons.
9. McKeown, 1965.
10. Department of Health and Social Security, 1976.
11. Gregg and Appleton, 1999, point out, however, that by 1994, 364 community paediatricians also recommended by Court were in post and that a further recommendation, that each district should have a handicap team, has also been accepted. They note that other countries are unfamiliar with the notion of community paediatrics in the British sense.
12. MACA, 1999.

13. Maggs-Rapport *et al.*, 1998.
14. NHS Executive, 2000c.
15. We consider this further in Chapter Five.
16. National Association of Health Authorities and Trusts, 1993.
17. British Medical Association, Royal College of Physicians of London and Royal College of Surgeons of England, 1998.
18. Royal College of Surgeons and British Orthopaedic Association, 2000.
19. In a health care system such as the NHS, a distinction can be made between the pattern of care delivery in terms of where things get done, and the management of that care. In the case of elective care, for example, the current situation in the UK is one of decentralised responsibility gradually being overlaid by central direction. It could be that the elective care system will shortly be a centrally managed system, run to standard rules, at least for some parts of it, e.g. those dealing with procedures such as CABG. The case for proceeding in this way is based on equity and not economies of scale or specialisation. Whereas in the US, many care providers are privately owned, multiple ownership can occur, thus reducing the number of care systems in organisational terms, but whether that influences the geographical pattern of service delivery is a separate matter.
20. This point is made very clearly in NHS Wales, 2000, and Standing Medical Advisory Committee, 1997.
21. This point is made in Harrison's (1998) review of the Calman/Hine proposals for cancer care.
22. Against the background developed here, the general hospital can be seen as a series of pathways that converge in geographical space and, usually, within the same management structure and often within the same professionals and facilities. Within the community, some pathways similarly converge in the GP practice or primary care centre, but others may converge in the homes of individuals, for a brief period of time, or more or less permanently. Against this background, the role of the management of hospitals, whether discharged by clinicians or non clinicians, is to help negotiate the various system interfaces. Although the evidence cited in Chapter Two suggests that this task is not carried out effectively, the formal structure of hospitals – and the current NHS organisational form of the trust – provides in principle at least a means of taking into account the interactions between care systems. In other words, the core role of the hospital management could be seen as that of reconciling the different claims made upon its physical and human resources. Outside the hospital there is no clear locus for this role within providers of care. Taking the health care delivery system as a whole, however, no such mechanism exists. Accordingly, if care systems are to be developed to include all contributing providers, then new mechanisms may be required (we turn to these in later chapters).
23. Mulligan, 2000b.
24. See Harrison, 1997.

25. Weiner, 2000; see also Shortell and Kaluzny, 1997, p 12. They suggest that health care has no characteristics unique to it, but that it embodies all the characteristics that make service management and delivery difficult in any sector.

Chapter Five

Professional roles and the structure of health care systems

If we were to continue with the 'thought experiment' set out at the beginning of Chapter One, then the process of determining the roles of the professionals would begin with the users or potential users of the health care delivery system, and proceed through the identification of how users needs would best be met, then the systems of care and the supporting services required, and from these to the skills and training of the workforce required to deliver the specified care. In other words, once the 'best' set of care systems was defined, the professional roles would themselves be defined in relation to them. As we have seen in the previous chapter, that process would be far from easy, but at the level of principle it would be the right one to choose.

But, despite the repeated protestations that the NHS should 'put patients first', in practice the way that services are organised and delivered, as well as the overall structure of the UK health care delivery system, reflects professional definition of care roles and the rules – including statutory limits on professional roles, accreditation by the professions themselves, or conventions arising from historical developments – that govern the contributions of professionals to the provision of care.

Of these many influences, perhaps the single most important is the nature and extent of clinical specialisation, since specialties define both the number and nature of the routes and pathways within the whole delivery system, as well as the services from which each care system draws. How they have come about is considered in the first part of the chapter.

While the division of roles between professions reflects a range of political and sociological factors, the extent of specialisation within each profession can largely be attributed to the growth in clinical knowledge over the past 100 years. Whether this process has gone too far, or not far enough, has mainly been considered in relation to each part of the health care delivery system. From the viewpoint of the whole delivery system, the key issue is whether the gains within any one system of care have been achieved only at the expense of imposing greater costs on others. This question is considered in the next part of the chapter.

We then return to the thought experiment set out in Chapter One, and consider its practical implications. If we acknowledge that, even as a thought experiment, it is impossible to take a clear view of the future, the question then arises as to how the training of professionals, which is extended in time and largely takes place at the beginning of their professional careers, should be linked into the development of systems of care.

As we have argued elsewhere,[1] clinical roles have largely been defined in terms of the effective delivery of particular interventions. The development of systems of care switches the emphasis from these to the context in which they take place, which places new demands on professionals. The final section considers some of the new roles that systems of care require.

How the system has been shaped

We described in Chapter Two the attempts of policy-makers over the years to find the 'best' organisational and financial structures for the NHS. Arguably, however, professional structures, largely uninfluenced by the policy of governments, have been much more significant in determining how the whole care system actually works. This process is not fully documented[2] and has not been uniform even within the UK.

Because, as we have seen, the NHS has never had a 'masterplan' setting out an overall delivery system divided into systems of care, the process of determining the roles of different specialties and the change in the balance between generalist and specialist hospital doctors has taken place at different speeds and in different ways in different hospitals.

One result is that no two hospitals work in the same way. As Holt[3] has put it:

> *There are over 250 acute hospitals in the UK and every one runs its clinical services in a different way. Differences may be slight or major but it is true to say that no two hospitals run in the same way. Each hospital has its own 'culture' and organisational environment. Organisation and management of clinical services is an area where NHS 'management' have historically had little input and abrogated responsibility to the medical profession at large.* (p 99)

Although the same specialty labels crop up more or less universally, their content varies. So the same condition may be treated under different specialties, or users may reach the 'right' specialty by different routes. Similarly, different hospitals have different arrangements for providing emergency care, particularly in the way that the 'take' and on-call cover is organised for medical and surgical emergency admissions. Equally, different specialties have different ways of organising their elective workload and within each there are variations between hospitals and even individual consultants.[4]

The variations Holt records reflect a persistent neglect of what appears to the patient to be the main function of the hospital – the response to an urgent need for care. Although the concept of the A&E department headed by a consultant is now established across the whole of the hospital system, it took a long time to do so: the first appointment of this kind was made as late as 1972, in part because of professional resistance to the notion that it could form the basis of a specialty.[5]

Although A&E is now established as a specialty, this has not resulted in a situation where the emergency care overall is regarded as a system of care, taking the whole of the health care delivery system or even the hospital. The emergency response function in hospitals is provided by clinicians who have responsibilities to other systems of care, and 'emergency' itself has not been the basis of a specialty exclusively dealing with all such needs.

We set out in Chapter Three the general arguments for considering 'emergency' as the basis for a system of care. Those arguments have had particular relevance in recent years in respect of acute hospitals that have appeared unable to cope at times of peak demand. The response, in local health economies urged on by the Centre, has been a series of attempts to create a system of emergency care from existing providers. Although that strategy has been partially successful,[6] the underlying issue of whether the professional and provider roles as they exist provide the most appropriate basis for such a care system has largely been neglected.[7]

The majority of emergency admissions do not need access to sub-specialist skills,[8] but there are very few medical consultants who do not practise one. One answer, therefore, as a report from the Royal College of Physicians[9] on the roles of specialists and generalists within hospitals concluded, is to make 'emergency' a specialty by introducing:

> ... *a new type of physician specialising in emergency care, whose duties might include running an admission ward, providing immediate medical care, assigning appropriate patients directly to specialties and supervising the initial hospital stay of the others*. (p 21)

Essentially, the same issues arise within surgery, where a similar solution has been proposed.[10,11] Outside hospitals, the response to emergency has also lacked a clear focus. As Coates and Goode[12] have pointed out:

> *In the UK there has been little medical interest in pre-hospital care, except by the general practitioners who volunteer to take part in the British Association of Immediate Care Schemes. The UK has only two consultant appointments in pre-hospital care within the National Health Service, and only one training scheme for specialist registrars that provides a structured education in pre-hospital care*. (p 1292)

Within general practice, the development of out-of-hours co-operatives in recent years has taken place largely as a result of local response to the rising number of night calls. It has not formed part of a systematic development of an immediate response system based in the community.[13]

The ambulance service apart, the provision of emergency care outside hospitals has attracted very little attention at national level for most of the life of the NHS. As we argued elsewhere,[14] because emergency care has not been treated as a distinct system of care in its own right, there has been no locus – no single professional group or organisation[15] concerned with how it worked as a whole and how it should be adapted in the light of new knowledge and new opportunities. More recently, as Nichol and Munro[16] have pointed out, the picture has become even more complicated with the introduction of minor injuries clinics, walk-in centres and NHS Direct, as well as the further development of out-of-hours co-operatives. All these appear to be separate initiatives with no clear indication as to how they should relate to each other.[17]

The development of geriatrics illustrates some of the same issues.[18] Its initial development as a specialty was in part fuelled by the belief of a small number of clinicians that unless it achieved that status, standards of care for the elderly would remain low. But that development had to fight against established views of what was medically important and what the basis of a specialty should be.

According to Isaacs: [19]

> *Much of the expertise of the geriatric physician comes from the recognition of recurring patterns of disability, the interaction between physical, mental and social factors; the intelligent and flexible use of the pool of resources; and the maintenance of mutual understanding between the many professional groups involved. To understand and to control all this requires much training and experience; and your mature geriatrician is master of many skills.* (p 226)

Furthermore, the prevalence of multiple morbidity challenged the basis on which specialisation has developed.[20] According to McCormack and Ford:

> *Doctors working with older people were considered inferior in status and skills, particularly as cure was the highly valued ultimate goal of the medical model. Older people do not fit easily into the standard medical paradigm A single diagnosis is rarely possible as disease manifestations are likely to be multiple and complicated by the effects of the ageing process. Add to this the social situations, social networks and an ageist society and one begins to see why working with older people is the challenge that it is. The 'quick cure' of one disease with no consideration of motivation, home circumstances and abilities is not possible.* (p 42)

The expertise of the geriatrician therefore comprises not so much command over a particular body of clinical knowledge as the ability to bring together the relevant knowledge from a number of areas and combine it effectively to meet the needs of a particular patient – in our terms, managing, as well as contributing to, a system of care.

Geriatrics is now well established as a specialty[21] (though the boundaries between it and general medicine continue to be contentious), but it too has not developed into an actual 'system of care', despite the fact that care for the elderly has been typified by failures of the various elements to be brought effectively together.[22] Here again the hospital/community divide has proved a major obstacle to developing services for the elderly that genuinely integrate all the individual service components, particularly at the boundaries between medical and social care and also within institutional nursing and residential homes, which fall between hospital and community responsibilities. The resulting gaps in provision have at long last been recognised and the process of (re)developing intermediate facilities begun.[23] But, as with emergency care, the issue of professional roles and their proper relationship to each other remains unresolved.

One critical failure has been the neglect of rehabilitation. The 1962 Hospital Plan envisaged that all hospitals would contain rehabilitation facilities, but the response was inadequate and patchy. When the Audit Commission[24] surveyed these services nearly 40 years later, it found that few hospitals organised rehabilitation services well.

Unlike emergency care, our analysis suggests that rehabilitation would not form a system of care in its own right. Instead, it should be a service contributing to all or nearly all systems of care. Its low level of development reflects its position as a supporting service, and also the nature of its knowledge base. As with geriatrics, a key component of rehabilitation is the *organisation* of the appropriate interventions.[25] According to Wade and de Jong:

> *Advances in rehabilitation contrast dramatically with advances in all other medical areas. The advances have occurred in service delivery; no important advances in single treatments have occurred. Consequently, it has been much more difficult for rehabilitation services to maintain or increase their share of resources in the face of expensive but effective single treatment advances in other fields*. (p 1388)

For many years, the King's Fund and other non-clinical organisations, as well as individual clinicians, have argued that rehabilitation services ought to have an established place in the NHS repertoire.[26] The NHS Plan envisages a large expansion of intensive rehabilitation services within hospitals and recuperation facilities outside them (para 7.4). That such proposals are now considered necessary reflects the failure of the unmanaged processes of specialisation, combined with a division of responsibilities and finance between different organisations, to provide what many of the systems of care based on other specialties actually require.

In the case of both emergency and geriatric care, the definition of a specialty has emerged because of a perception on the part of some clinicians that specific needs were not being well addressed by the existing set of specialties. But that achievement remains a partial one since it is has not led to the development, in practice, of systems of care comprising all the relevant providers. As a result, the notion of a system of care remains in both cases essentially an analytic one.

Next, we take two instances – the relief of chronic pain and low vision services – where the professional response to user needs has been slow, with the result that in some cases no service has been provided at all. As far as pain services are concerned, Wall[27] notes:

> *Medical, dental and veterinary schools were set up to purvey the principles of their profession. The cause of disease and fundamental cures were the main target. Symptoms such as pain were mere signposts on the road to the main aim. Symptom control was historically not worthy of the attention of serious men so this task was assigned to denizens of the depths of the hierarchy, such as nurses and physiotherapists. Even dying was not a worthy subject because, by general medical agreement, there was nothing more to be done.* (p 167)

Against this background, it is not surprising that services to provide relief have had to struggle to establish themselves. The Clinical Standards Advisory Group found in a report[28] published in 2000, but reflecting conditions a little earlier, that:

> *A low priority was accorded to chronic and acute pain services by the majority of both Health Authority and GP commissioners. This view was not shared by hospital staff and a minority of GPs and was not generally based on an assessment of patients' wishes or needs.* (p 21)

The report adds:

> *Most Health Authorities supported the provision of an acute pain service in principle but were not involved in achieving the provision of such service. Most perceived the funding of acute pain services as an overhead to surgery. Many GPs were not aware of acute pain services, did not see the need for a service, and did not wish to pay any extra cost for its provision, and felt provision was the responsibility of the Trust. Neither group attached a significant added value to the provision of such a service.* (p 21)

As a consequence, patient needs were neglected; their opinions on 'added value' were not canvassed. One result, as Wall records, has been a substantial growth of self-help groups.

The second example comes from low vision services. People with poor vision, for whom surgery is unable to help, can nevertheless benefit from professional support. But such support is patchy and provided in a large variety of ways by a large variety of professionals, none of which has made it its own area of expertise. According to a recent survey: [29]

> *Professionals within low vision teams referred people to one or more of 31 different types of agency or professionals [table 5]. There appeared to be no uniformity in the number or nature of links that a low vision service provider had and in general the provider type did not predict the links a provider had.* (p 22)

This finding reflects a failure, as with pain services, for the 'naturally' developed professional structures to recognise a user need. In this case, the need 'belongs' to an existing specialty – ophthalmology – but that specialty has not seen it as part of its remit to meet it.

These two examples are the tip of a large iceberg of services that have been overlooked.[31,32] As with pain relief, in many cases this has been compensated for by the creation of self-help groups or by voluntary bodies, and in some cases their work has led to the gaps being filled, or funding has been obtained for the organisations themselves to fill them.[32] In the present context, they serve to illustrate the way that professionally defined roles may not match up to patient needs at both the system of care level and the level of the individual component.

In principle, the policy innovations described in Chapter Two, particularly the development of national service frameworks, should reduce the mismatch between provision and need. But, as we shall see in the next section, there are further issues to be resolved before that conclusion can be reached.

The limits to specialisation

We have argued that the process of specialisation within the medical and other parts of the workforce has been the main force for structuring the care pathways by which patients access care. That process has been largely unregulated and unplanned and, as the examples considered above suggest, has not always produced an effective delivery system. In other areas such as cancer or cardiology, the process has, in general, been assumed to be so obviously beneficial that it needs no justification. Nevertheless, it has not gone unchallenged, both on clinical grounds and also because of its wider impact on how the health system works.

As far as the first of these is concerned, there is considerable professional and research literature that supports clinical specialisation. This literature has been surveyed by the University of York in a series of publications[33] and, while their general conclusion is that the advantages of medical and surgical specialisation have been overstated, the evidence does not suggest they do not exist. The issue, rather, is where the threshold at which those benefits become small or disappear lies.

While the York review remains the best available overview of the benefits of specialisation as measured by scale of activity,[34] it did not consider whether the basis of specialisation in current clinical practice is appropriate. Indeed, given the nature of most of the evidence available, it could not be, since nearly all of it is based on individual specialties or even individual procedures, and the search for benefits confined to each one in turn.

In other words, the benefits of specialisation have been identified 'locally', that is to say that the studies concerned have focused on particular procedures or activities and have not, in general, sought to identify any costs in the health care delivery system as a whole that such specialisation might give rise to. However, the framework of analysis developed in previous chapters suggests such costs may arise in several ways.

First, patients may not fit the boxes or there may not be an appropriate box. The prime reason for the former is co-morbidity. According to Schellevis,[35] there are four types of co-morbidity (see Box 5.1 below). Particularly important in the present context is category (c), since that may determine the nature of the skills required and determine the form of treatment used for any one.

Box 5.1 The nature of co-morbidity

(a) *concurrent co-morbidity*: the co-existence of diseases in the same person without any satisfying explanation, e.g. cardiovascular disease and osteoarthritis;

(b) *cluster co-morbidity*: the distribution of diseases in a population shows concentrations in sub-groups that differ significantly from the distribution by chance, e.g. multiple sclerosis and epilepsy;

(c) *causal co-morbidity*: interrelation of diseases based on a proven common pathophysiological cause, e.g. ischemic heart disease and peripheral arterial disease;

(d) *disease-specific complicating co-morbidity*: the existence of one disease is obligatory for the occurrence of another disease, e.g. diabetes mellitus and diabetic retinopathy.

Source: Schellivis, 1993.

Taking the user view, it is clearly important, whatever the type of co-morbidity,[36] to have the range of conditions they suffer from addressed at the same time by one person, or team, competent to consider all of them. In the words of a report by the Royal College of Physicians: [37]

> *4.24 … Patients dislike being cared for by several different specialists if they have more than one condition and would prefer their care to be the prime responsibility of a single physician whom they know and trust, but who also has access to advice from other specialists as necessary. This is as true for secondary specialist care as for primary care.* (p 23)

The report adds:

> *There is little firm evidence about whether they have a better outcome when they are treated by a specialist physician or a generalist. Apart from acute asthma, it is unclear whether outcomes are any different when patients are managed by specialists or general physicians in collaboration with the specialists (31–34). In this context it is worth noting that there is a rapid retreat from multiple specialist care in the United States where the need to contain costs is driving care in the direction of the general internist.* (p 23)

As things currently stand, however, users suffering from co-morbidities may, above all other categories of user, find their pathways to be long and fractured, in part because they do not 'belong' to one specialty box and in part because the process of obtaining all the relevant clinical information may be long and arduous and involve a series of visits to the same hospital or diagnostic centre.[38]

The development of geriatrics can be seen as one response to this phenomenon, since co-morbidity is common among the elderly. But it is not confined to them. There is very little information available[39] about the reasons for multiple hospital visits, in particular whether these reflect attempts to find the right 'specialty box' or to combine inputs from different boxes. However, the greater the number of specialty boxes, the larger the group of patients who do not fit any one is likely to be and hence the chances of their pathway being complex or not well defined all the greater.

Second, specialisation across the full range of clinical disciplines may make the overall delivery of care less efficient, even if it makes for greater efficiency within each, particularly where clinicians continue to work in more than one care system – that defined by their area of special knowledge and the emergency system.

According to Taylor:[40]

> ... *excessive specialization inevitably results in individuals losing skills, which could inhibit their ability to remain on the hospital emergency rota. If a surgeon spends too much of his working practice in breast disease, for example, he may lose the skills associated with abdominal surgery, and hence be unable to provide a comprehensive emergency service for trauma.* (p ii)

If they did not have the dual function, the issue would, of course, not arise.

From the viewpoint of any one system of care, its definition and management is made easier if resources are specific to each pathway. That may mean both more specialisation between care systems and less within each of them. The first will occur when some professionals focus purely on a task or specific care group; much of the development of nursing specialties[41] reflects developments of this sort. The second arises when resources are trained to do a wide range of tasks along a pathway or within a system of care. Both tend to reduce calls on shared resources.

But one result of this process may be a reduction in the overall efficiency of the whole health care delivery system. In a review of the workforce requirement of the NHS, the HSMU report[42] argued that the costs of specialisation across all clinical work had been underplayed. The fragmentation of the workforce that existing job definitions embodied produced:

- *problems in the provision of cross-cover;*
- *inflexibilities in responding to peaks and troughs in workload;*
- *lack of clarity of accountability;*
- *increased delays and confusion for patients;*
- *wasted time as staff wait for completion of work by other occupations;*
- *increased time spent in coordination and meetings.* (p 6)

These points suggest that it would be beneficial to create less specific human resources that can readily be transferred along and between systems of care.[43] The need to provide for such flexibility stems in part from the unpredictability of the clinical workload in the short and longer term.

In the short term, the need arises particularly in respect of emergency care and variations in demand from hour to hour and day to day, etc. Most UK hospitals provide that flexibility by transferring nurses from one part of the hospital to another, but both medical and surgical specialists may also transfer. This implies an across-the-board capability among most clinical staff. However, this approach also means that the unpredictable emergency side of the hospital persistently imposes costs on the predictable planned side.[44]

In the longer term, the need for flexibility rests on the growth of clinical knowledge and the impossibility of forecasting what form it will take. As the King's Fund evidence to the Health Committee inquiry into NHS workforce planning[45] put it:

> ... *future workforce requirements are inherently difficult to predict in the light of major uncertainties about the future pattern of health care demand and service delivery; hence flexibility is required in training programmes and staffing arrangements*. (p 347)

Professional training is long and expensive, and represents a large personal and social investment. Against a background of continuing growth in clinical knowledge as well as social change, it represents a risky investment. In some areas, the 'need' for a particular specialty may decline – as has been the case recently with gynaecology – or the technology on which it is based may alter, making old knowledge and techniques obsolete.

The ability to predict such changes is very limited, as is understanding of how specialist roles have changed in the past. As one of the many committees[46] tasked with forecasting the 'need' for doctors, commented:

> ... *the pattern of health care delivery has changed, as one would expect with the increased use of sophisticated technology and machinery, but it is not possible to tell from the statistical data available whether the professional and technical staff took over work which would otherwise have been done by doctors or whether they were needed to implement technological advances which complemented the doctors' work*. (p 25)

This was written 20 years ago, but the same conclusion would be reached now, as the pace of technological change has shown no signs of diminishing. The implications for the nature and degree of specialisation have yet to be full grasped.[47]

The overall balance

If we accept that we have now, or can define in principle, the set of specialist and generalist clinical categories required to answer the question posed in our thought experiment, then the balance between the various 'clinical knowledge bundles' would emerge as an outcome of that process.

That process has not been applied to the health care delivery system as a whole. Instead, there has been extensive discussion of the balance between specialists and generalists as broad categories, particularly in those countries which consider that their generalist, community-based service is weak. In the US, for example, many commentators, of which Starfield[48] has been perhaps the most prominent, have argued the case for a system of general practice along the lines of that within the NHS and other European countries, while others[49] have bemoaned the 'over-emphasis' on specialists:

> *There is widespread concern, however, that despite the benefits of biomedical science and medical professionalism, the US health care system is precariously off balance. A model of excellence focused on specialization, technology, and curative medicine has led to relative inattention to basic primary care services, including such needs as disease prevention and supportive care for patients with chronic and incurable ailments.* (p 167)

But where is the line between over-emphasis and balance to be found? If we were to return to our thought experiment, in the absence of a system of care by system of care approach, how would we determine the division of clinical, primarily medical workforces between hospital and community?

This question has been addressed implicitly by workforce planning committee after workforce planning committee. It has rarely, if ever, been addressed explicitly, through a consideration of the benefits of deploying varying amounts of the various bundles of medical knowledge that the existing array of specialties including the generalists embody. Instead, each specialty has made claims for more and has been more or less successful in the process.

The role of the Centre appears to be little better discharged. The NHS Plan, for example, simply asserts how the expected increase in medical workforce will be split between general practice and specialists, but no justification is offered for the proposed division and indeed there is no agreed analytic framework available for doing so.

As we will note in Chapter Eight, attempts have been made at very aggregate levels to determine whether the balance between generalist/community and hospital/specialist is right, by comparing health outcomes between countries with high and low proportions of their medical staff in specialist and generalist roles. But this work is of little help in a system like the NHS, where the community generalist is well established and where the issue is whether or not to expand that role in its present form or to develop alternatives such as nurse practitioners.

The framework developed here does not provide an answer, but it leads to a re-framing of the issue. As we have argued in Chapter Three, it is unhelpful to argue for the expansion of 'primary care' in general, as its content is so unspecific. It is more helpful to consider which elements of which systems of care can and should be provided in a local context. This in turn might lead, as noted in Chapter Four, to a modification of the way the generalist role is discharged through, for example, the development of local specialists, or it may simply continue the trend established for some time for parts of the hospital workload to move into the community, in response to technical developments such as new drugs and monitoring devices that allow community professionals or the users themselves to take on new responsibilities.

New roles

Alongside specialty definitions, the definition of professional roles has been critically important to the structure of health care delivery. Like the development of specialties, the current 'system rules' are best explained in historical terms.[50] These rules bear on two main questions – 'who does what?' and 'who can decide what?' across the Service as a whole.

The first of these has attracted a great deal of attention as a result of economic pressures and the shortages of particular categories of staff. Many hospitals, for example, have been forced by the shortage of junior doctors resulting from the (belated) policy of reducing their working hours to use other staff in their roles.[51] Outside and inside the hospital, there has been a vast range of experimentation with different skill mixes.[52] We noted in Chapter Two the experiments in the local delivery of general practitioner services, which include the substitution of nurses. Nurse prescribing, which was officially endorsed some 20 years ago, has gradually come to be accepted and is now, in the NHS Plan, fully supported.[53]

While the question of who does what is clearly important when considering the efficiency with which services are provided, it is the second question – who can decide what?, i.e. the extent of professional discretion – that is more important for the definition and design of systems of care.

While specialisation had been the main force shaping health care delivery during the twentieth century, towards the end of it another trend came into play, the spread of discretion to more and more professionals. At the turn of the nineteenth century, the nurse was clearly the handmaiden of the hospital doctor and the division of role virtually absolute, but soon after, a long drawn out process became apparent by which nurses, particularly in hospitals, plugged the gaps left between medical specialties. By the beginning of the twenty-first century, many nurses and other professionals had acquired room for independent action and clinical responsibility, and could be regarded as 'specialists' in their own right.[54]

These developments are important in the present context because the number of pathways – or routes within a care system – is critically dependent on the nature of discretion allowed to specific clinicians. In general, the health care system has been run like a chess game, in which the medical staff are the queens, capable of any (legal) move, while the rest are highly constrained pawns with little room for independent action. This has meant that nearly all care pathways have had to 'run through' a doctor, in hospital or the community, when a decision to move the patient along the pathway had to be made. These constraints are now being substantially relaxed, in the process opening up opportunities for new, shorter and hopefully quicker pathways.

In some contexts the process of relaxing the constraints on professional roles has had little impact on the care pathway itself. In many hospitals the discharge decision has become a nursing role: delegation of the discharge decision has allowed the patient to move more rapidly along essentially the same pathway. But, in other contexts, the growth of discretion has led to the development of new pathways. In the case of emergency care, routing discretion is not normally granted to the ambulance service: its staff have had little scope either to provide treatment or to determine which hospital to take a patient to. But, where time is critical, allowing discretion to ambulance staff can be vital to a successful outcome. As one study[55] found:

> *All experimental models, and clinical trial experience with thrombolysis in stroke, suggests early treatment is critical in maximising benefit; a principle encapsulated in the phrase 'time is brain'. Acute-stroke assessment by paramedics may be sufficiently accurate to permit redirection of patients to centres with acute-stroke units.* (p 1935)

Within hospitals, the main routing decisions have largely been the preserve of doctors but, as already noted, the decision to transfer the patient to another setting is now often made by nurses. The introduction of triage nurses at the entry to the hospital has varied from the trivial to the fundamental in terms of its impact on how the A&E department functions. However, extension of this triage role can, like the ambulance example just cited, create new and shorter pathways. It may, for example, lead to patients being returned to a community setting without entering hospital at all, provided that suitable community-based services, particularly rapid response home-based support, are available.

In the community, the decision to refer to specialist advice lies almost entirely with general practitioners. However, there are others who exercise similar discretion over the routing of patient, although they do so relatively rarely. As Craig[56] has pointed out:

> *... community clinical medical officers refer patients to paediatric and eye clinics, health visitors can refer to hearing clinics, eye clinics or child psychiatry, orthoptists refer to eye clinics, social workers can refer to child psychiatry and some consultants allow patients to re-refer themselves to outpatient clinicians.* (p 82)

These sources of referral are not identified or even recorded in official statistics (e.g. of waiting times to access hospital specialists), but they are, probably, of growing importance. In some areas, new referral routes are being developed on a trial basis.[57] But, in the case of maternity care and mental health, they are already fundamental to the way the service works. In respect of the latter, GPs are far from being the important referral source, as Table 5.1 indicates.

Table 5.1 Referral source: mental illness

Referral Source	*Number*	%
Casualty	32	28
Outpatients/domiciliary visit/CMHT	39	34
IHTT	12	10
Psychiatric ward/hospital	10	9
GP	7	6
Police	5	4
Social services/voluntary agencies/other	10	9

N = 115; Missing = 35

Source: Godfrey and Williams, 1998.

Both community midwives and community mental health nurses act as independent agents in their own clinical practice and themselves determine when specialist medical support is required. The NHS Plan envisages extension of such discretionary roles:

> *NHS employers will be required to empower appropriate qualified nurses, midwives and therapists to undertake a wider range of clinical tasks including the right to make and receive referrals, admit and discharge patients, order investigations and diagnostic tests, run clinics and prescribe drugs.* (para 9.5)

The extension of discretion allows the delivery of care to be more responsive to users because forms of delivery can be envisaged outside the traditional hierarchy of control. Thus, minor injury units run by nurses have developed,[58] operating, like nurse prescribers, within defined limits and able to provide a local service close to patients, and thereby counter the forces making for the centralisation of emergency care facilities in larger units. The same is true, as noted in respect of open access schemes,[59] of the roles of different types of medical staff.

These examples illustrate the general point that the growth of specialisation and the spread of discretion leads to the health care delivery system becoming more complex through the creation of more connections between clinicians and more routes for users to travel along. But, as the number of routes and hence the number of pathways increases, the knowledge required to utilise and manage it may lag behind.[60] As a result, the potential of the improved pathways may not be realised. We noted above GPs lack of knowledge of pain relief services. There are other examples. An Audit Commission report[61] on the case of sick children found:

> *... largely historic referral patterns which can result in routine conditions being treated at expensive regional centres, while more complex surgery is attempted at district level.* (p 25)

Another study[62] found that, where a hospital had created a fast track for AMI admissions, a large proportion of GPs was not using it because they needed to do so only rarely and were therefore unfamiliar with the procedures to be followed.

One response to growing complexity in the referral role is the introduction of referral advisers to general practice – another example of the unbundling process described in Chapter Three. Another response is the explicit mapping through referral guidelines of the range of pathways that are open and their suitability for particular groups of patient. McColl *et al.*[63] report there is support within general practice for action in three areas:

> *First there was general support for the production of directories of hospital services. These could include basic data about the services available, staffs' special interests and procedures for referrals, admissions and domiciliary visits ... Secondly, general practitioners expressed a desire for an opportunity to take part in a defined programme of observation in selected hospital clinics ... Thirdly, the use of the term urgent in referral communications is a fruitful topic for audit and educational activities. A multidisciplinary task group might usefully develop an agreed set of guidelines for the general (or specific) use of the term and how consultants act upon its use.*

The first two of these in particular can be seen as a response to a growing number of referral ways that has created a need for a more systematic approach to the provision of information and informal learning.

Another response is the creation of new roles. The critical contribution of the definition of pathways is that the process provides the context for the work of the individual professional, as his or her work is seen as one contribution to the care of the patient representing only part of a much longer sequence of care. The same applies to the broader concept of the system of care.

As indicated above in respect of emergency services and older people, professional as well as organisational barriers have been important obstacles to the development of effective care systems. As things currently stand, the answer to the question 'who is in charge?' is 'no one'. As a result, certain elements of care systems receive virtually no attention at all.

This is particularly true of services that lie at the margin of the hospital and the community. One such is outpatient services. A report from the National Patient Access Team[64] found that most of the hospitals visited had not changed their systems for managing outpatients (of which there were many) for decades, despite the standards set in the *Patient's Charter* nearly a decade before. Similar, repeated failures[65] have been recorded at the discharge end of the hospitals' role.

In recognition of failures of the second kind, a range of new roles has developed, such as that of discharge nurse and care co-ordinator.[66] The first is aimed at improving a particular and notoriously difficult interface, the second at the broader task of ensuring that all the elements required by an individual are in place.

The notion of a pathway suggests a sequence of events, the one leading to another – the patient journey. In some cases, however, the key professional task is to ensure the simultaneous contribution of different professionals as well as to harmonise these contributions over a period of time. This role is identical to that which within the social care field goes under the name of care or case management (Box 5.2).

Box 5.2 Case management

Case management is a system of care delivery that focuses on the achievement of outcomes within specified time frames and efficient use of resources. Hospital-based case management approaches tend to parallel the discharge planning process in the assessment, identification of needs, planning specific actions, and the coordination of services. It differs from discharge planning in that some models of case management cross all settings in which the patient receives care.

Source: Bull, 2000, p 72.

As the extract indicates, the notion of case management arises from the need to ensure that the various elements in the pathway are defined and in place, and that the patient receives them in the appropriate order and at the appropriate time.

These developments have important implications for the training of health care professionals. The pathway and the system of care perspective runs counter to the traditional form of medical and other clinical training, as well as much of the research literature, which is focused on the individual intervention, the specific professional role or the process of care within a relatively narrow ambit such as a ward, operating theatre or GP practice.

The logic of the pathway and the system of care is that the clinical horizon for most practitioners should be wider, extending beyond whatever is their area of professional competence to encompass the broader context in which they work. Some may continue in their traditional roles, but others must take on the new ones that arise from that broader perspective. But exactly what these should be depends critically on the way that pathways, programmes and systems of care

are defined, in particular whether, as suggested in Chapter Four, they cut across the deep-seated boundaries between hospital and community.

Conclusion

The development of professional roles over the past 100 years can be seen as a sustained process of specialisation, leading to ever more routes for patient journeys and more systems of care. As a result, the health care system as a whole has become more complex, offering more routes, more elements of care along those routes, and more interconnections.

The gradual development of job contents, new roles and modification of training represent the same process as that described earlier in the chapter – the piecemeal adaptation of the workforce to new perceptions of how clinical work should be organised and carried out. Most of the technical innovations involved in the definition of care pathways have been aimed at making the current structure work better, in some cases by making changes in the distribution between professionals of the elements in a care pathway. But, in general, they have not questioned the underlying structure itself, particularly the definition of the professions. But, if the Service was to be designed from scratch, these too would come into play.

If the work of professionals is to be defined by reference to 'user needs', then we require a clear idea of what these comprise. In practice, we have only a limited ability to assess what those needs are, both now and in the future. Assuming these *were* established, following the logic of the argument in the previous chapter, the next step would require resolution of the series of choices involved in determining what the structure of service delivery should be: how many systems of care there should be; on what basis they should be determined; how they should relate to each other; how users should be routed into them; and how independent of each other they should be. As these questions were resolved, definitions of professional roles would follow.

In practice, these questions have never been tackled simultaneously with the benefit of an overall view, but rather in a series of largely independent developments driven by a number of different factors, of which only some could be said to be 'user needs'. The incremental process can be effective, particularly as we cannot be confident enough in our abilities to forecast the future to set out a single vision of the future pattern of health care delivery to form the basis of new definition of professional roles. But that lack of confidence fits badly with the form that professional training takes, i.e. a large upfront investment spread over many years. This, like investment in fixed assets such as hospitals, is risky. Although the need for continuous clinical training has been recognised, the main emphasis continues to be on the initial stage of the process.

A final challenge comes from another direction. Much of the knowledge that defines the notion of a professional is now readily available through a wide range of media. The next chapter considers the implications of this development for the way that professional roles are discharged.

References

1. Harrison and Dixon, 2000, Chapters 8 and 11.
2. See, for example, Stevens, 1980 and 1996, and Rosen, 1949.
3. Holt, 1999. Holt goes on to point out that UK hospitals manage emergency admissions in several ways and their comparative merits have not been evaluated.
4. This is apparent from the reports of National Patient Access Team: see, for example, Department of Health, 2000h.
5. For reasons that might now seem odd. In the paper 'Orthopaedics', in Craft *et al.*, 1975, Vickers puts the argument as follows:

   The arguments against the specialty are first, the lack of continuity of patient care. This argument could also be levelled against the large specialties of anaesthetics and pathology, and is invalid. Any consultant is at liberty to follow up his own special interests in his field and, in casualty, the field is wide open. The second argument is that no one worthwhile would enter this field because it is not rewarding. This argument is about as valid as an orthopaedic surgeon saying that he does not know why people wish to carry out prostatectomies (p 25).
6. NHS Executive, 2000b.
7. See, however, Chapter Seven below, where this issue is further considered, and Coffey and Mythern, 2000.
8. Hampton and Gray, 1998, point out that:

   The specialist can offer a package of management that allows patients to gain maximum benefit from a team best fitted to deal with their particular – usually continuing – problem. Some patients admitted as emergencies clearly require such a package, but many do not and few require it on the day of admission. It would be inappropriate for the physician running an admissions ward to see it as his or her function simply to sort the patients into the care of the 'apparently' relevant specialist: where treatment is properly evidence based (as, for example, in the care of patients with acute myocardial infarction), management is by protocol that can be followed by any physician, or indeed by appropriately trained nurses. The patients who might benefit most from specialists are those whose optimal management remains undefined: for example, all those admitted with ischaemic chest pain without infarction ('unstable angina') could fit into this category, but the number of patients involved and the expense of handling all of them through a single-specialist system would make this model of care impracticable. (p 42)

9. Royal College of Physicians, 1996.
10. This is suggested in Loefler, 2000.
11. See also Mainous *et al.*, 2000, who put forward the notion of what they term a hospitalist who would provide general medical care to non-surgical patients.
12. Coats and Goode, 1999.
13. See, however, the report on out-of-hours services published in October 2000: Department of Health 2000i.
14. Harrison, 1997.
15. Arguably, the ambulance service does, but it has never been in a position to be the integrating agency across all the other contributors to emergency care.
16. Nichol and Munro, 2000.
17. We return to this issue in Chapter Seven.
18. See, for example, Grimley Evans, 1997, who points out that in most countries geriatric medicine has yet to develop.
19. Isaacs, 1981.
20. McCormack and Ford, 1999.
21. But not in all countries. Furthermore, as with emergency care, there is a range of models as to how geriatrics is and should be practised: see Black and Bowman, 1997.
22. See, for example, Audit Commission, 1997a, and Millard, 1991.
23. The NHS Plan proposed a significant growth in such facilities.
24. Audit Commission, 2000b.
25. Wade and de Jong, 2000. They conclude that: 'Rehabilitation has started to become an evidence-based specialty.'
26. Nocon and Baldwin, 1998.
27. Wall, 1999. The Audit Commission report on pain services (Audit Commission, 1997) points out that many patients 'endure a long search – often over many years – around different parts of the NHS and the private sector seeking respite prior to their arrival in a chronic pain clinic' (p 84).
28. Clinical Standards Advisory Group, 2000.
29. Ryan and Culham, 1999.
30. Davis *et al.*, 2000, point out that chronic disease can be seen as a field of inquiry in its own right, but neglect in the past has meant that the knowledge base is poor, even for common conditions such as asthma.
31. The NHS Cancer Plan (NHS Executive, 2000c) points out that only a third of health authorities has developed strategies for specialist palliative care.
32. We look at this further in the following chapter, but see in particular Mackenzie, 1979, and Wood, 2000, who give many more examples.
33. Ferguson *et al.*, 1997.
34. See also Donehoe, 1998, who takes a much broader approach.
35. Schellevis, 1993.
36. See Wagner, 1996, particularly p 532, for a discussion of the significance of comorbidity for service design. Coebergh *et al.*, 1999, provide data on the incidence of

co-morbidity among cancer patients. In Birmingham, a service for people with epilepsy and a learning disability was established in 1997 in the face of an almost complete lack of research on this combination of conditions.

37. Royal College of Physicians, 1996.
38. A joint report from the Royal College of Physicians and Royal College of Psychiatrists, 1995, notes that:

    Although common, psychological disorders may not be recognised and adequately dealt with in the general hospital. This is because (a) many interviews fail to elicit psychological problems, (b) modern medicine is orientated towards technological investigations which may divert attention away from psychological problems, and (c) many staff have not received adequate training or encouragement to pay sufficient attention to the psychological aspects of patient care. Such training and encouragement require the support of a liaison psychiatry team (psychiatrist, liaison nurses, social worker and psychologist) who must be readily available and appropriately skilled to provide rapid and comprehensive treatment when necessary. (p 1)
39. Their importance can be inferred from the large number of inter-consultant referrals.
40. Taylor, 1997.
41. See Armstrong, 1999, and Ibbotson, 1999, for reviews of the development of nurse specialists.
42. Health Services Management Unit, 1996.
43. This point has formed part of the case for the development of generic care workers: see, for example, Anderson, 1997.
44. See discussion in Chapter Four.
45. House of Commons 1999b, Appendix 68.
46. Medical Manpower Steering Group, 1980.
47. The growth of continuing medical education has been one response.
48. Starfield, 1994.
49. Grumbach and Bodenheimer, 1995.
50. See, for example, Parry and Parry, 1976, Rafferty *et al.*, 1997, and Rafferty, 1996.
51. McKee and Black, 1991.
52. See Jenkins-Clarke *et al.*, 1997, for a review.
53. It was announced in autumn 2000 that 10,000 nurses were be trained in prescribing.
54. See Armstrong, 1999, and Ibbotson, 1999.
55. Harbison *et al.*, 1999.
56. Craig, 1996.
57. Robert and Stevens, 1997, concluded that:

    The studies included in this review suggest that there are several advantages for patients who are referred directly for physical therapy (either to an open-access physiotherapy department or to a physical therapist attached to a GP practice). The main advantages are the significant reductions in waiting times, convenience, and reduced costs for the patient and also the health authority in terms of cost per treated patient. There is also some evidence that the recovery time may be slightly better for patients who receive direct-access physiotherapy. (p 317)

58. Salmon *et al.*, 2000.
59. Davies, 1999.
60. On the other hand, the creation of new routes, e.g. through direct access schemes, may enable GPs to make better routing decisions to hospital specialists.
61. Audit Commission, 1999b.
62. Thomas *et al.*, 1997.
63. McColl and Hutchinson, 1994.
64. Department of Health, 2000h.
65. Marks, 1994.
66. See, for example, Nazarko, 1998.

Chapter Six

Users and systems of care

Our thought experiment began, in Chapter One, with a simple statement of what characteristics an ideal health care system would have, from the user's viewpoint. But up to this point we have focused almost entirely on the professional considerations that have shaped the way that health care delivery system functions. Even though the care pathways discussed above refer to individuals, in most definitions of pathways the individuals themselves are typically treated as passive objects rather than decision-makers in their own right.

That in turn reflects the assumption that has typified most discussion of health care systems, that the user is poorly informed relative to the professional, and hence the professional is 'in charge'. Indeed, it is this information imbalance that underlies the very notion of professionalism and the paternalism that goes with it.

This imbalance is beginning to change in response to:

- the growth in availability of information about medical conditions
- the growing importance of chronic disease, which means that a larger number of patients live with their conditions for long periods of time, come to know them well and have first-hand and unique experience of the impact of different forms of treatment on them.

Acknowledging these developments, the White Paper *Saving Lives: Our Healthier Nation*[1] put forward the notion of the 'expert patient', recognising that many people with chronic conditions effectively knew more about those conditions, at least as they affect themselves, than their professional advisers:

> 3.49 *People with chronic illnesses are often in the best position to know how to cope. There is increasing evidence from research studies and from patients' associations that people have improved health and reduced incapacity if they take the lead themselves in managing their chronic disease – with good support from the health service.* (p 39)

Furthermore, the growth of knowledge bearing on the delivery of care poses difficulties for professionals themselves, making it ever harder to bring all the available knowledge to bear on the clinical problems that users present.[2]

The rise of the 'expert patient' has obvious implications for the clinical encounter, when users and professionals meet to determine the appropriate pathway and how, if it all, the user should progress along it. The implications for the broad structure of health care delivery are less obvious. The link between the broad structure, i.e. the division of the whole health care delivery system into systems of care, organisations and professional roles and the quality of care provided, is indirect and not easily perceived by the individual patient. While some features such as access, both in physical and availability terms, are readily perceived, the implications of providing good access on the quality or cost of the service are not. Furthermore, while users can and do have views as to the nature of the care they are seeking, these views may not be identical. As with any other service, different people may place different values on different characteristics with, as noted at the end of the Chapter Four, different implications for the structure of service delivery.

Moreover, while 'services are for users', other considerations come into play, principally the needs of professionals as workers. While users might want 24-hour availability of services and continuity of care with the same individual professional, that combination cannot easily be reconciled with the needs of professionals themselves for rest and recuperation, training and other personal needs. And in health care systems, where access costs are zero in money terms, some means must be deployed to reconcile the resources available with the demands users place upon them.

This chapter begins by extending the analytic framework set out in Chapters Three and Four to take users explicitly into account, by introducing the *informal* care system that complements the formal, professionally delivered, care system. We then go on to consider a number of relationships between the two. Next we consider the role of demand management in influencing the way that users approach and enter into the formal system. In the final part we look at the potential for redesigning the formal system to better meet user requirements.

An analytic framework

All care pathways start with the individual seeking something from the health care delivery system and the system exists to meet or try to meet the need identified. The traditional assumption has been that, at this stage, the nature of the required response is unknown. Hence, the primary function of the front-line health care service is to sort or route the patient to the most appropriate part of the whole system. That process may be immediate or long-winded. It may lead to a single encounter or a sequence of care events and decisions along a care pathway.

In most examples of pathways defined in practice, the patient is 'in the system' and the task of the care providers is to design an efficient pathway and then ensure that the patient proceeds down it and its various branches as quickly as possible. In the models of health systems set out above, we included users as the first element in each care pathway and in Figure 3.3 explicitly identified the scope for users to opt out or change course.

The scope for independent decision is most obvious right at start of the care pathway, where users decide whether or not to seek professional help. It is 30 years since Julian Tudor Hart[3] wrote about the concept of the clinical iceberg – suggesting that patients who demand care represent only the tip of the iceberg of need, as illustrated in Figure 6.1 below:

Figure 6.1 is often used to illustrate the differences between need, demand and use.

Figure 6.1 The clinical iceberg of disease

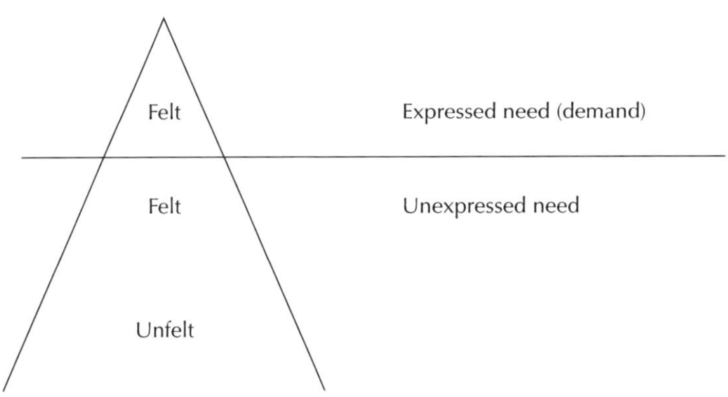

The iceberg analogy implies that there is more unexpressed than expressed need. Hence, most 'need' in the population does not come to the attention of those providing care within the formal system. When patients actually express their need as demand by presenting themselves to a GP or to A&E, that demand in turn may not result in service use if the professionals concerned decide it is inappropriate to provide a response.

Figure 6.2 Need, demand and use

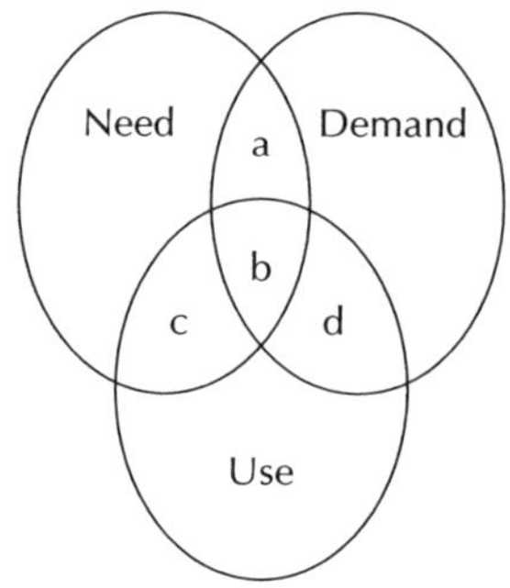

Note: Area (a) illustrates the case where care is needed and demanded but not provided by the NHS, for example care that may no longer be available on the NHS such as cosmetic surgery. Area (b) indicates that care can be needed, demanded and utilised, for example patients undergoing effective elective surgery. Area (c) indicates that care can be needed and utilised but not necessarily demanded, for example routine immunisation or population screening for cervical cancer, which people must be actively encouraged to use (and some do not). Area (d) indicates that care can be demanded and provided but not needed, for example antibiotic treatment of viral infection.

Of the four areas shown in the diagram, area (b) is the least controversial: this is the area that any effective health care delivery system will supply. Area (a) embodies a conflict between what users want and what the system provides: any health care delivery system must embody such an area if it is maintain control over its budget. Whether it is appropriately defined or not is largely a political question, at least within a publicly funded system such as the NHS, of what care should be offered free of charge. Where control is exercised through means other than price, then it embodies a conflict between, on the one hand, the freedom of the individual to choose and, on the other, broader social arguments that suggest freedom to choose might not be in their own or the overall interest.

There is a further way of defining the content of area (a). As noted in Chapter Five, there are some services that 'should' be provided, but which do not fit the existing professional structures: chronic pain control, palliative care and rehabilitation are all areas that have had to fight for inclusion within the formal system, in large measure because the professionals did not view these functions as what a health service should consist of.

Area (c) reflects the point made above, that users are free not to use a service. But another interpretation of this area is the way in which the Service is configured, and the extent to which its existence is adequately explained or publicised (in the appropriate language, for example) may be such as to deter use. The existence of wide variations in access to some elective treatment cited in Chapter Two arises, in part, for reasons like these.

The final area, (d), reflects 'bad' decision-making on the part of a professional. But it may also reflect a difference between the user's view of what should be done and the professional's view of what is an appropriate response to a perceived need. The professional may offer something, perhaps an antibiotic or a placebo, simply to handle this conflict in an acceptable way.[4]

The formal and the informal system

Although Figure 6.2 is helpful in setting out some of the key relationships between user and system, it omits a key feature – the scope for self-care. Potential users have always dealt with a vast range of problems themselves, relying on their own judgement or that of family and friends, and their knowledge of the effectiveness of drugs they can buy over the counter.

As Table 6.1 shows, the vast majority of 'incidents' are dealt with by people without resort to professional help. Quite small changes within the informal system can have significant implications for the formal system, because of the disparities in their relative sizes.

Table 6.1 Responses to minor ailments

	Children	*Adults*
Saw doctor or dentist	17%	13%
Used a prescription medicine already in the house	13%	13%
Used an OTC medicine	33%	24%
Used a home remedy	11%	9%
Did not use anything	28%	45%

Source: BMRB, 1997.

If we include self-care, the whole care delivery system, in simplified form, looks like this:

Informal System + Formal System = Whole System

But this simplifies the relationship between the formal and the informal. As Tudor Hart has also argued,[5] the user is a co-producer of care, even if professionals have been reluctant to acknowledge this.

> *Even doctors who regard all patients as passive and uncomprehending consumers of their skills, limit history-taking to cross-examination, and confine treatment to unexplained prescription or referral, must in all circumstances except acute emergencies depend on patients' participation and co-operation in their own care.* (p 383)

The 'capacity to produce care' is partly a matter of informal or formal programmes of 'instruction', such as chronic disease self-management programmes[6] designed to support the self-care system. It also depends on the wide range of factors that influence the individual's capacity to deal with disease.

Although this capacity is a basic physiological characteristic and is reflected for example in the placebo effect, what determines it and how it may be strengthened is not well established.[7] In practice, more emphasis has been put on the changing nature of the relationship between user and professional. The term 'patient partnership' has started to come into use to describe the relationship between the formal and informal system arising from the increasing knowledge available to, and now being exploited by, users (see Box 6.1).

Box 6.1 Patient partnership

This appeared as a priority in the *NHS Priorities and Planning Guidelines* for 1996/97 and was explained as follows:

- *appropriate and effective services are more likely to be developed if they are planned on the basis of needs identified in conjunction with users;*
- *growing social expectations of openness and accountability mean that the users of public services are increasingly seeking more say in how the NHS is developed, what services are provided and to what standards;*
- *patients want more information about their health condition, treatment and care. The Patient's Charter responded to this trend by formally stating a right to such information, but it is of course integral to the whole notion of 'informed consent';*
- *there is some evidence that involving patients in their own care improves health care outcomes and increases patient satisfaction;*
- *as we become gradually more sophisticated in assessing clinical effectiveness and outcomes, it is important to find ways of communicating that information to patients in a form they can understand and to ensure that the information itself reflects the patient's perspective on the benefits of their treatment.*

Source: Department of Health, 1997, p 3.

The points in Box 6.1 apply all along the care pathway, not simply at the point of entry into the formal system. Accordingly, the relationship between the informal and formal system is better described by Figure 6.4.

This diagram embodies three main features:

- the interaction between the formal and informal system is continuous
- the patient is partly in charge of whether or not to proceed along the care pathway
- the patient is also a producer of health care.

If we were designing a formal health care delivery system from scratch, how would it take account of these points? As far as the structure of care is concerned, the key analytic point is the disaggregation of the function of first contact services into the components of advice and care. Typically, they have been combined within one person, e.g. a general practitioner. But increasingly the roles are becoming distinct, with the development of telephone advice from GP practices and A&E departments through to the national system of NHS Direct. The advice may be to use the formal system but equally it may not: as Box 6.2 indicates, NHS Direct appears overall to be diverting very few demands away from the formal system.

Figure 6.3 Combining the physician and patient models

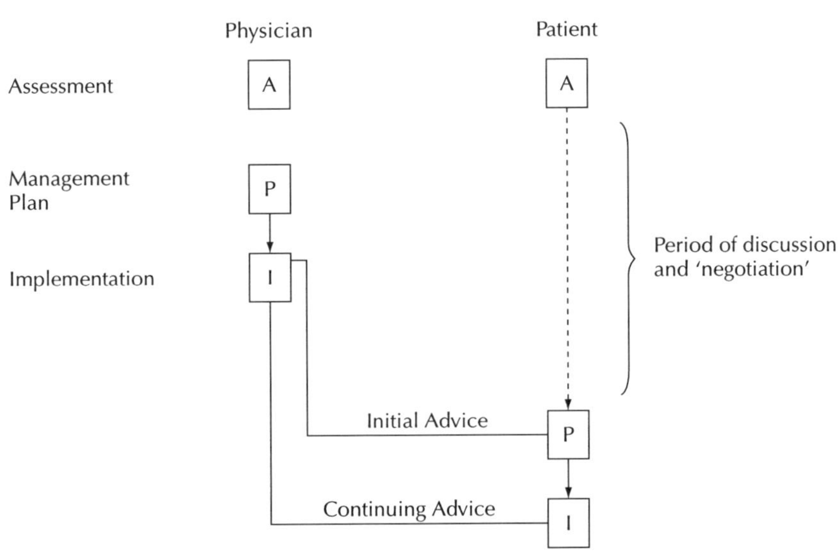

Within the informal system itself, the critical resource requirement is knowledge in the form that potential users can assimilate. Where once such knowledge was scarce, it is now available in excess. The critical additional requirement is, therefore, its quality. NHS Online implicitly provides such quality assurance, as do the many other information sources provided by reputable organisations worldwide.[9]

Although these sources can be valuable, they are not the main route by which patients become 'experts'. Those who do, do so on the basis of their own experience or that of others close to them or with whom they are in contact through self-help groups. As we shall note below, development of this form of expertise may lead beyond a simple reduction of user reliance on professionals to structural change in the way that care is delivered.

Box 6.2 NHS Direct

The introduction of a national scheme of telephone advice, NHS Direct, might have been expected to encourage a switch from the formal to the informal system. However, the early results of the monitoring of NHS Direct[8] suggest that it has had limited impact on overall use of the formal system. According to the University of Sheffield monitoring report:

... it is perhaps surprising to see from the charts and figures in this section that the thousands of calls to NHS Direct each month are not having more visible impact on overall demand for immediate care services. The impression rather, is that NHS Direct contacts have simply been added in to the overall picture of health service use for unplanned health care problems. It is possible that NHS Direct has improved the appropriateness *of demand for services without having a great impact on* total *demand, although the stability of 'least urgent' demand for A&E and ambulance services suggests that such an effect could not be a large one.* (pp 65–6)

The implication is that its main benefits may lie in improving the efficiency of the informal system, i.e. the effectiveness of self-treatment – but no provision was made for monitoring this, no doubt because self-care remains a largely implicit system of care, with little formal recognition.

A further key factor is the availability of the other resources a user may require for self-care. Among these, the most commonly available is over-the-counter medicine, but they may also include access to testing and diagnostic equipment. In the case of diabetes, for example, self-monitoring of blood sugar levels is now the norm, if not universal.

But users must have confidence that what they are doing by themselves is 'safe'. The present system does not always provide this assurance. As the Audit Commission report on diabetes services noted,[10] a substantial proportion of the patients they surveyed had received no advice in the previous 12 months and many did not have the knowledge or the confidence to manage their condition.

Finally, although personal knowledge and the way that services are provided are important determinants of the scope for self-care, other key factors determining it lie elsewhere, particularly in personal and social attitudes towards acceptable risks and the perceived value of what professionals have to offer. For professionals, the issue of risk is a delicate one, linked as it is to the potential for negligence claims. In practice, professionals themselves had largely decided what risks were acceptable. That is beginning to change, with implications, as we note below, for system design.

In conclusion, to term self-care a system of care in its own right may seem an exercise purely in re-badging the familiar. It is, however, perhaps more than that. As with emergency care, recognition by national and local policy-makers that it is, in analytic and real-life terms, a system of care, could lead to new forms of service provision and the commissioning of relevant research designed to make it more effective.[11] New services might include specialist advisers for those with chronic conditions, paralleling similar developments for GPs.[12] As for research, self-care does not feature in the areas defined for research in recent R&D policy documents, but it clearly should, if only for the reason given above – that it is potentially cost-saving.[13,14]

Managing demand: entry to the formal system

The previous section suggested that the scope for self-care may, among many other factors, influence the manner and the extent of use of the formal system. In this section we consider in more detail the interface between the formal and the informal system.

Guiding entry

The NHS has for most of its life been passive – accepting, in effect, the patient's decision whether or not to approach the Service, and not giving the potential user much guidance about whether or not to use it or which part of it to approach. The situation now is radically different. The introduction of NHS Direct means that decisions on both can be taken on an informed basis.

So far, the evidence suggests that access decisions can be improved, since the early monitoring results[15] found that users' original intentions to access the formal system or a particular part of it were modified by the advice they received.[16]

Table 6.2 Comparison of expectation with advice given

	Expectation			
Advice	*A&E Dept* %	*GP immediately %*	*GP in next few days %*	*Self-care only* %
A&E dept	57	13	10	14
See a GP immediately	12	50	20	13
See a GP in next few days	11	28	57	21
Self-care only	15	8	15	46
Total = 100%	131	120	112	269

Source: Munro *et al.*, 1998.

Controlling entry

The main structural rule governing access to the NHS is that users cannot approach specialists directly. This restriction rests on a number of assumptions:

- people do not know what is wrong with them and hence they cannot rationally select a specialist
- if they do know what is wrong, they do not know whether or not they need a specialist
- even though some patients may be well informed some of the time, there is no way of determining when they are
- if unrestricted access is allowed, the result will be inefficient in terms of the use of specialists' time.

Although the existence of this rule is normally called gatekeeping, in our analysis it is better described as 'routing' – the GP determines not only that the patient may proceed beyond the gate but also determines the appropriate entry point to specialist services, other hospital facilities such as diagnosis, or to community-based services such as chiropody, speech therapy or osteopathy.

As we have noted in Chapter Four, there are some long-standing exceptions to this. In the case of eye and dental services, users are assumed to know where to go and to be able make their own choices as to which entry point to use, a situation that has existed since the foundation of the NHS. In other areas, where restriction has been the norm, the rules of access are beginning to change in large measure in response to the development of the expert patient, whether formally recognised or not. A report from the Long Term Medical Conditions Alliance,[17] for example, found that:

> *Most hospital out patient services dealing with inflammatory bowel disorders in particular will now offer patients self-referral. This means that patients who have a chronic disease are seen at minimum necessary follow-up intervals, usually once or twice per year. In some clinics, patients will now have a direct access telephone number to either contact a consultant, clinical research fellow, or gastroenterology nurse experienced in dealing with their problems.* (p 7)

A related option is for the first-line contact itself to be more specialised than the GP. As noted in the previous chapter, that model already exists for some community services, particularly mental health, and it could be generalised to other conditions, particularly those of a chronic nature.[18]

Access to emergency care has never been controlled; the assumption has been that the user can make a judgement as to whether his or her condition justifies immediate access – in effect, allowing the patient to be 'expert'. In practice, surveys of the use of A&E services have persistently found that many users are seeking convenient as much as immediate access. Furthermore, the rapid increase in the use of ambulances as well as A&E departments in recent years suggests that the convenience factor is becoming more significant in decisions as to how to access emergency care.

As the increase does not apparently reflect any increase in morbidity or the frequency of accidents, it has led to calls for some form of entry control. As NHS Direct is currently operated, it provides only advice. But it might be used as an entry control device, following the pattern adopted within some managed care schemes in the USA. As Salisbury has suggested, '... NHS Direct could become the *only* way into the system'.[19]

Salisbury notes there would be some risks with this, but it would be the route towards developing a unified system of emergency care. A more attractive approach from the user angle would be to signpost the emergency care system better, a task that a unified system of care would find it easier to do since the roles of the various elements would be more clearly delineated. Such a system might include new pathways, avoiding the use of hospitals made possible by better triage within A&E departments and a wider availability of urgent response teams in the community.[20]

Promoting entry

In most circumstances, publicly financed health systems do not actively seek users, i.e. do not attempt to convert need – area (a) – into utilisation: the assumption is that the user can be relied upon to decide if he or she needs professional help. But use may be actively encouraged on a sporadic basis, where there are outbreaks of infectious disease such as meningitis, and on a regular basis, where there is a case for immunisation and vaccination, as with children, and screening for specific diseases such as breast cancer in adults.

The encouragement may be justified both by the direct benefits to individuals and the indirect ones (which the individual may not take account of) through the creation of group immunity. The introduction of call and recall screening programmes implicitly assumes that the 'normal' process of presentation does not work adequately because some women may present too late for the treatment to have much chance of success. In the case of breast cancer, however, in recent years part of the gain in life expectancy is attributable to earlier presentation. That may be due to the introduction of a formal process for calling women for mammograms or to earlier identification by women themselves,[21] which itself may be encouraged by 'breast awareness' campaigns.

In other areas, use is encouraged by eliminating the normal barriers, e.g. through open access clinics for GUMs, which avoid the possibly embarrassing visits to a GP. In these circumstances, the user may be assumed to benefit directly, but there may also be a benefit to the system as a whole if improved access now reduces future utilisation, either by the users of such facilities themselves or those they might infect.

Managing use

As our analytic framework and the subsequent discussion of the scope for self-care indicated, the underlying need and the recognised need may be influenced directly through measures taken to prepare users for dealing with incidents of ill health themselves. Equally, such measures may be used to increase service use by helping patients to identify the need for professional care. These measures we term 'demand management': they act both to increase and decrease the numbers of users deciding to access the formal system.

In addition, health care delivery systems must also embody measures to manage utilisation. Within the formal system, many uncodified rules or informal, even personal, strategies influence the way that care pathways work, most importantly the extent to which professionals can demand resources on the part of their patients. Codified rules such as protocols and referral guidelines may also have this effect, where they do in fact impact on professional behaviour.

Though formal and informal rules are important in determining how demand for care is matched on a day-by-day basis with the resources available to meet it, the design of systems of care has a role to play. In the case of emergency care, the appropriate response may be a combination of triage and the creation of low-cost routes that divert users away from A&E departments, such as minor injuries units, more intermediate post-operative care or better support at home, as well as support for self-care, as discussed above. It is probably easier to divert users to lower-cost forms of care than to limit their access.

From the viewpoint of the system of care, all forms of demand and utilisation management must be considered as a whole and must be regarded as part of the

Box 6.3 Definition of terms

By 'demand management' we refer to measures taken to influence the decision to use the formal care system. These might be long-term preventive or promotional measures or short-term measures, such as the provision of information or advice in paper or electronic forms.

By 'utilisation management' we refer to measures that influence the service actually used. This includes long-term measures, such as system design to ensure an appropriate range of options is available and day-to-day measures, such as GP gatekeeping or telephone advice or triage.

definition of the care system. And in both cases, there is a need to take into account the possible response of users and professionals to a change in system design. To demonstrate this, we take the example of waiting lists for elective care.

In the case of elective care, the NHS has deployed the full range of rationing strategies, but the most prominent has been that of delay. From the system viewpoint, this is a useful attribute since it helps to bring demand into line with the available supply. But whether this deterrent effect is desirable turns on what exactly is deterred, i.e. whether minor conditions that may not require urgent treatment or indeed treatment at all, or whether people are put off presenting more serious conditions by the expectation that they will have to wait for treatment. Although the existence of a deterrent effect is supported by a number of studies,[22] its precise role is far from clear.

Over the years, successive governments have aimed to reduce the numbers waiting and the longest waits, but despite success as far as maximum waits are concerned, only very limited progress has been made as far as numbers waiting. Both users and professionals have responded to the changes made and in effect reversed them.

Now, in the NHS Plan, the present government has set out its intention to reduce waiting times to substantially below their current level. If waits are required to bring the demand for and supply of elective care into balance, and if waiting times are reduced, balance can be restored only by the introduction of another form of access control, such as thresholds or referral guidelines[23] – unless the supply of elective care is increased. In other words, if one demand management tool is relaxed, another form of control must be brought into use, unless sufficient extra resources are introduced to produce a new balance between demand and supply at a sufficiently higher level of activity to meet the extra demand ensuing as a result of the relaxation of control.

From the user angle, no form of control is welcome. But if control is to be exercised, what would be its preferred form? As we have argued elsewhere,[24] following developments in New Zealand,[25] the nature of the control or threshold ought to be both explicit and based on acceptable principles.[26] This requirement is essentially a political one, but in a publicly funded system such as the NHS, there is a close link between how the Service as a whole is regarded and what individual users see as being acceptable. The present government has acknowledged this in one important respect, by making improved and more convenient access a specific objective.[27] It has yet to take the step of explicitly acknowledging that, despite the massive increases in resources that the Service is now enjoying, there remains a limit on what it can provide.

Users and the design of systems of care

Most of the desirable characteristics of a health care delivery system set out in Chapter One are not closely linked to the way that systems of care are designed and delivered. Any system of care should embody them. Furthermore, as we noted in Chapter Three, defined pathways have value in themselves to users, giving them reassurance that they are progressing, irrespective of their value in defining professional roles. And other familiar features of the current pattern of provision – the existence of a geographically dispersed system of general practice and local general hospitals – have always been promoted on the grounds of easy access as well as, in the former case, the continuity of care that registration with a selected GP has been assumed to offer.

In themselves, these features are not contentious; the difficulties arise only when their preservation is put at risk by other changes designed to 'improve care for patients'. Where, as with the gradual closure of smaller hospitals in favour of larger ones, access may have to be traded for quality of outcome, different users would make that choice differently. In practice, they can have only one or the other. In some cases, however, choice may be available, as the example of maternity care shows.

Whereas maternity care was once largely based at home, in the post-war period the locus shifted to hospitals and home births virtually ceased. From the 1970s onwards, there was pressure from users and from some professional groups, particularly midwives, to reverse that trend. The issues and the opposing viewpoints were examined by the Health Committee of the House of Commons in 1992.[28] Its report came down heavily on the side of greater choice, i.e. a system of care that offered alternative care pathways. A subsequent report, *Changing Childbirth*[29] endorsed that position and it was subsequently adopted as official policy.

Leaving issues of professional power to one side, the differences between the two sides of the argument lay in the areas of risk and continuity of carer. The hospital-based professionals argued that safety was paramount and that, as hospitals could cope with all contingencies, they were the best location. Others argued for the management of risk through patient selection and back-up through flying squads to deal with emergencies so as to allow other values, of which continuity of carer as well as a degree of user autonomy were the most significant.

In this example, user pressure has led to the redesign of a system of care. In other areas, users may identify gaps in provision. In the case of pain relief, for example, Wall[30] comments as follows on the response to the failure of the formal system to supply a service:

> *The situation I have described leaves a scattered, invisible underground population of people seriously disabled by their ongoing pain and yet abandoned and ignored. It is not surprising, in this situation, that self-help groups spring up all over the world as patients revolt at their neglect.* (p 172)

These groups may and do develop their own collective expertise. More than 20 years ago, Mackenzie[31] noted the development of groups representing patient interests. A more recent review[32] charted their rapid development. Since then, using the Internet and other media, they have provided an alternative source of advice to the formal system and may, through their own form of specialisation, exceed it in depth of knowledge. The result may be that the patient begins to teach the professional.[33]

These examples suggest that the definition and design of health care systems is too important to be left to the professional system itself. This leads to the question: would the overall structure be radically different if scope for the development of the informal system and users' views of the formal system were taken into account more systematically?

It seems unlikely that, with existing technology, the main structural features of health care delivery, particularly the hospital and the local health centre containing general practitioner and related skills, would disappear. But both the nature of the clinical relationship and the care pathways faced by users could be very different if the role of patient as expert and as producer of care was further developed. The frontline would consist of more advisers and routers, and fewer carers. This might involve, as noted above, the development of direct access pharmaceutical advice for patients as well as professionals, particularly for those receiving multiple medication. More fundamentally, it might lead to new professional roles, independent of the existing bundles of expertise, focused on advice and support across a range of disciplines. The core skill would be the effective transfer of knowledge, rather than the possession of one particular form of knowledge.

More radically, if the notion of the expert patient was further developed so as to allow direct access to specialists and if the professional organisation of care in community setting came to be built around care groups, as outlined in the previous chapter, then the system would present a wider range of routes than currently exists (at least in the NHS).

But going down this road is far from straightforward, even from the user angle. The creation of new routes giving direct access to specialists might suit some, but others (or the same people in different situations) might prefer continuity of care – a generalist role. Similarly some may prefer easier access, but others may trade that off if they have continuity from the same carer (or, again, the same people may make different choices in different situations).[34] Despite the large amount of work that has been done to ascertain 'user views', little of the evidence bears on these and other structural features.

Conclusion

We have argued that self-care can be regarded as a system of care in its own right, which can be supported by provision of information and by changes in the way that the formal system is configured and in the rules under which it operates. It may also be enlarged by the provision of formal 'courses' in self-management. In these ways, the boundary between informal and formal systems and the role of the formal system may be altered.[35,36]

We have also indicated that taking user views into account may lead to the design of specific systems of care and the introduction of new elements to existing ones.[37] Whether the overall structure of the health care delivery system – the definition of systems of care, the roles of different professions and the links between both of these and formal organisations – would be different if user views were more consistently taken into account is less obvious.

First, in most circumstances it is not clear how changes in the structure of health care delivery will change the various characteristics important to users. As the previous chapter made clear, some of the key relationships between different structures and health outcomes are not well understood.

Second, even if these were clear, how users would value those characteristics relative to each other is also unknown, as is the scope for offering, within the NHS, choice between different ways of delivering care within one system.[38] These considerations argue for experiment with new service designs on the one hand, and more systematic research into user preferences and their relative valuation of different service characteristics on the other. Although the NHS has begun a systematic survey process[39] of its users, it has not yet embarked on systematic research of user preferences for different forms of service delivery at the broad strategic level that has concerned us here.

References

1. Secretary of State for Health, 1999.
2. Weed, 1997, but also McKeown, 1965.
3. Tudor Hart, 1995.
4. Dixon and Sweeney, 2000.
5. Tudor Hart, 1995.
6. See, for example, Wagner *et al.*, 2000, and Wagner, 2000.
7. As Dixon and Sweeney, 2000, have pointed out, the potential for cost saving it represents should by itself suggest that a substantial research effort was worthwhile.
8. Munro *et al.*, 2000.
9. One example is the Johns Hopkins site: www.jhu.edu
10. Audit Commission, 2000a.
11. See Holman and Lorig, 2000, who describe or refer to several self-management programmes, and Clark and Gong, 2000.
12. See Dennis and Owens, 2000, and Audit Commission, 2000a, which sets out a programme of patient education.
13. Department of Health, 2000e, 2000f.
14. But it may be valued for other reasons as well, not least the pleasure of not being reliant on others.
15. Munro *et al.*, 1998.
16. Towards the end of 2000, the present government launched a campaign designed to make people aware of the options open to them – to use the pharmacy or the advice line instead of the GP. This in itself indicates that the entry points to the formal system are not clear or well understood.
17. Long Term Medical Conditions Alliance, 1999.
18. Dennis and Owens, 2000.
19. Salisbury in Salisbury *et al.*, 1999.
20. As suggested, for example, in the national service framework for mental health and official advice on the management of winter pressures.
21. Miller *et al.*, 2000.
22. Harrison and New, 2000.
23. The National Institute for Clinical Excellence has begun a substantial programme defining referral criteria for a range of conditions.
24. Harrison and New, 2000.
25. Hadorn and Holmes, 1997.
26. The author took part in a Channel 4 *Despatches* programme (23 November 2000) on waiting for care, which clearly demonstrated, through case studies, the lack of any such explicit principles in the management of NHS waiting lists.
27. See NHS Plan, para 1.1.

28. House of Commons Health Committee, 1992.
29. Cumberlege, 1993.
30. Wall, 1999.
31. Mackenzie, 1979.
32. Wood, 2000.
33. As Muir Gray, 1999, has noted:

    The parent of a child with a rare metabolic disease who happens to have had a scientific education will be able to find, read, and understand a paper about the gene deletion in Nature*, whereas most clinicians would be out of their depth with such a paper. Furthermore, as patients learn that know-how is as important as knowledge and that many clinicians do not have the know-how of managing chronic disease, they will share know-how with one another.*
34. See Brampton, 2000, who makes a strong case for continuity of care – but also adds that she wants the back-up of specialists within a polyclinic – i.e. not as far away as the hospital.
35. Such a change may not, of course, be to the liking of those working in the formal system. As Bradley and Blenkinson, 1996, have noted, the development of self-medication:

    could split the professions as they squabble with the patient and each other for the last vestige of control of medicines, leaving the patient baffled, confused and vulnerable to the dangers inherent in all medicines taking. (p 837)

    Nevertheless, there are many signs that the nature of the clinical encounter, at least for some patients, is beginning to change in a way that offers the user greater control and autonomy.
36. Ferguson *et al.*, 1997.
37. Gutch, 2000, argues strongly, with examples, for the potential user role in service design.
38. The market answer to the question posed here is competition, but even a non-competitive NHS can offer choice between different modes, particularly where the competition comes from lower tech and cheaper forms of treatment.
39. Airey and Erens, 1999.

PART THREE

Policy implications

Chapter Seven

Systems of care and organisations

The picture that emerges from the discussion in the previous chapters is far from neat and tidy. In contrast to the simplicity of the hierarchy model, the structure of a total care delivery system as we have identified it comprises a number of overlapping and interdependent care systems, the scope of each based on different criteria, and a series of services typically defined by function or professional group, which sometimes fall entirely within the definition of one system of care and sometimes not.

So far, however, we have focused on systems of care as units of *analysis* and we have argued that at that level they have several merits. However, if systems of care are to have significance in the real world, they have to be embedded in specific institutions – what we termed 'formal organisations' in Chapter Two. These may be profit seeking firms or voluntary bodies seeking only to cover costs or, as in the NHS, they may be trusts subject to a demanding accountability regime, or general practices subject to a much less demanding regime but nevertheless one that shapes the manner of their operation. The central question we consider in this chapter is: how can systems of care and formal organisations fit together?

One answer, reflecting large areas of current practice, is that the relationships between clinicians can work, as noted in Chapter Five, in a kind of parallel universe, cutting through the formal barriers of organisations and working almost independently of them. The relationships between community and hospital-based clinicians are largely of this kind. They largely operate on an informal basis,[1] yet they represent one of the central structural features of the NHS. Similarly, within community-based services, working relationships between GPs and other professionals employed by trusts or other organisations may be closer than those between some of those working within the same formal organisation such as a hospital.

One answer, therefore, is that the essentially clinical relations of a system of care can co-exist within the essentially managerial relationships embodied in formal organisations. That is the answer implicit in recent policy developments. However, the formalisation of clinical procedures using protocols or guidelines leads, by reducing the discretion enjoyed by clinicians, to 'organised' behaviour, in the sense that it follows rules laid down in advance. In this way, the pathway may be more organised – in the sense of following explicit and generally accepted rules – than the organisations of which it forms part. This implies, as we suggest below, that it may be appropriate to consider groups of pathways or systems of care as organisations in a formal sense and to reconsider the nature and role of formal organisation as it exists now.

Furthermore, the development of care pathways and programmes of care such as national service frameworks involves strengthening not simply the day-to-day working links between professionals in different organisations: it also implies a shared responsibility among the participating clinicians for the quality of care on offer. As things currently stand, however, finance, contracts and arrangements for clinical governance are centred on the formal institutions of the NHS, principally trusts and general practices/primary care groups/primary care trusts, and health authorities. If systems of care do not respect these boundaries, the question arises as to whether the new arrangements are appropriately located within a set of formal organisations, the scope of which is defined by quite different criteria.

This chapter begins with professional networks and then considers the role of contracts. As noted above, the introduction of contracts between parts of the NHS, as well as between the NHS and the private sector, opened up the possibility of new forms of care delivery emerging while leaving the boundaries of formal organisation untouched. We then consider the scope for changing the boundaries of formal organisations to fit systems of care and then the value of formal organisation itself, in a whole system of health care delivery divided up into systems of care.

Professional networks

No health care delivery system can function effectively without the flow of information to and fro within informally or formally defined care pathways. Although information remains bottled up in individual organisations or parts of organisations, in principle it can, however, permeate the barriers created by organisational boundaries, and in practice it does so through the GP referral or the hospital discharge letter.[2] Communications of this sort arise from the movement of an individual patient along a care pathway.

The *definition* of a care pathway involves the exchange of information of a more general kind. As noted in Chapter Five, shared care and other ways of creating the conditions for effective working between professionals located in different institutions have largely been focused on protocols, guidelines, shared care and the formalisation of care pathways, etc., all of which tend to promote better and a more timely exchange of patient information across organisational boundaries. However, clinical integration requires agreed working procedures over who does what and what should be done in specific sets of circumstances. The information exchanged in the process of reaching such agreement may in principle involve all the relevant research evidence bearing on the particular pathway, as well as information relating to costs and staffing.

However, the formalisation of pathways or systems of care involves the exchange of information in a different sense. By defining who does what in what circumstances, formalisation influences the expectations of individual clinicians about their own roles and about how the system of which they form part will respond to the decisions they make. Where the formalisation of care pathways running across organisational boundaries succeeds in bringing about agreement on these central issues, it brings about the order that in other contexts it might seem only formal organisation could achieve.

At one level, clinical co-operation between non-competing public sector bodies such as trusts would seem clearly desirable, mirroring the professional networks that exist in private sector industries or the research community, even where the organisations involved are in competition for markets or for funds.[3]

However, the development of clinical networks rests on a further consideration. The key point as far as hospitals are concerned, already anticipated in Chapter Four, is that the clinical economics of each specialty or system of care require different catchment areas, and the more closely systems of care are defined the more this will become apparent. As the Standing Medical Advisory Committee[4] remarks:

> *The optimum size of population served by a system of care may vary for different patient groups and for different medical specialties*. (para 3.3)

As noted in Chapter Two, some of the studies carried out for the London Implementation Group argued for systems of care running across several hospitals for a number of care groups. These were based on the notion of hubs and spokes, the former being the more specialised or teaching and research hospitals, and the latter usually general hospitals.

'Hub and spoke' embodies at least two different concepts. The first is an essentially clinical arrangement between clinicians in different hospitals in different organisations, based on a shared understanding of who does what and who should be treated where: the second represents a single clinical team providing services in different hospitals.

This second model was developed by some (then) free-standing specialist trusts, in part to preserve their market position after the 1991 reforms. Many of these, however, have since been merged into larger units. However, the way of working they developed could be seen as foreshadowing the development of systems of care in their own right.

More recently, the Scottish Office *Acute Services Review*[5] argued that the 'hub and spoke' terminology implied a hierarchy, when partnerships between clinicians might be more appropriate. It therefore proposed what it termed the 'management clinical networks' we have already referred to. A subsequent circular, *Introduction of Managed Clinical Networks within the NHS in Scotland*,[6] elaborated the notion in the following terms:

> 45. *As an alternative to the 'hub and spoke' model, some of the networking systems described to the Review feature the sharing of patients, expertise and resources, rather than unidirectional centripetal flow ... The emphasis in clinical networking is on connection and partnership rather than isolation and self-sufficiency, on distribution of resources rather than centralisation, and on maximising the benefits for all patients rather than a fortunate few ... This model has significant implications for service management, particularly where networks have to develop across traditional boundaries such as those between Health Boards.*

As the final sentence acknowledges, clinical networks involve the transfer of clinical responsibility for patients and also resources from one organisation to another: hence, the way they work has implications for those organisations over and above the movement of patients through them. However, the circular appears reluctant to spell these out (see Box 7.1).

The measures set out in Box 7.1 are, in effect, intended to make the existing poorly organised parallel universes work better by making them more explicit as well as more important to the clinicians involved in them. But neither of the documents cited above is explicit about the links between the clinical connections and formal organisations between which they are made. The implications for the participating organisations are not examined.

Box 7.1 Clinical networking

8.1 each Network must have clarity about Network management arrangements, including the appointment of a person who is recognised as having overall responsibility for the operation of the Network, whether a lead clinician, a clinical manager or otherwise. Each Network should produce a written annual report to the appropriate Health Board or Trust, which would also be available to the public;

8.2 each Network must have a defined structure which sets out the points at which the service is to be delivered, and the connections between them;

8.3 each Network must have a clear statement of the specific clinical and service improvements which patients could expect as a result of the establishment of the Network;

8.4 each Network must use a documented evidence base, such as SIGN guidelines where these are available, and must be committed to expansion of the evidence base through appropriate R&D;

8.5 each Network must be truly multi-disciplinary/multi-professional and should include representation from patients' organisations in its management arrangements;

8.6 each Network must have a clear policy on the dissemination of information to patients, and the nature of that information, bearing in mind the role of primary care in helping to lead the patient through the system;

8.7 all the health professionals who would make up the Network must indicate their willingness to practice in accordance with the evidence base and with the general principles governing Networks;

8.8 an integral part of each Network must be a quality assurance programme acceptable to the Clinical Standards Board for Scotland, which also has a role in ensuring consistency of standards and quality of treatment across all Managed Clinical Networks;

8.9 the educational and training potential for Networks should be used to the full, through exchanges between those working in the community and primary care and those working in hospitals/specialist centres. Networks' potential to contribute to the development of the intermediate specialist concept should also be kept in mind, and Networks should develop appropriate affiliations to universities, the Colleges and SCPMDE;

8.10 all health professionals in the Network must produce audit data to required standards and participate in open review of results;

8.11 all Networks must include arrangements to circulate staff in ways which improve patient access, and enable professional skills to be maintained. Each Network should have an appropriate programme of continuous professional development in place for every member of the Network, as well as a mechanism for ensuring the programme is being followed;

8.12 there must be evidence that the potential for Networks to generate better value for money has been explored.

Instead, the Scottish Executive circular refers to 'virtual organisation' without attempting to define that term: it simply states:

> *Networks can therefore be characterised as 'virtual' service organisations, where the skills of the professionals concerned are grouped around the population and service needs and may not be co-terminous with Trust or Health Board boundaries*. (para 46)

Although the term 'virtual' is in wide use to describe how organised behaviour can occur between the boundaries of formal organisations, the term hides as much as it reveals about what is really intended. The circular recognises this and goes on to state that 'the concept of the lead clinician [is of] central importance' without elaborating what that means.

The issue the circular is trying to address in this indirect way is 'who is in charge' of a clinical network or system of care based on a disease or client group that extends beyond the boundaries of any one formal organisation. The issue is the harder to avoid the greater the commitment to developing a system of care across existing boundaries and the more it becomes the focus of other policies, particularly those relating to clinical governance.

As far as the first of these is concerned, the establishment and development of a system of care involves investment in new facilities as well as staffing, both of which imply financial commitment for the organisations contributing to the system of care. As far as the second is concerned, if, as for example the national service frameworks envisage, monitoring performance against defined standards is introduced, then issues of control and accountability will inevitably be pushed to the fore.[7]

In brief, the further a system of care moves from an analytic concept to a practical reality, the more it takes on the characteristics and roles of a formal organisation. How are the two to be reconciled? Essentially there are two main options: contractual and organisational integration.

Contractual integration

The notion of a hospital that emerges from our analysis is of an institution that:

- provides short episodes of care to longer care pathways
- contains conflicts in terms of competing claims on resources from different pathways.

Except where an A&E department provides a 'singleton' episode of care, the hospital as care provider is a contributor to a large number of more widely defined systems of care. The historical division between hospital and community has conspired to hide that. As we shall see below, however, progress can be made by re-conceptualising the hospital role in a way that could lead to change in its organisational form.

As already noted in Chapter Three, however, the case for using systems of care depends on a series of interdependencies between different providers or between support services. While formal organisation can internalise these by, for example, allowing for financial cost-shunting between care systems through internal accounting procedures, systems of care running across organisations can do so only if the flow of funds through contracts can allow for these interdependencies. Recent innovations in the financial framework applying both within the NHS and between the NHS and local authorities' social care services open the way for 'financial treaties' between organisations that reflect their interdependence. Thus, in principle, cost shunting and benefit spillovers can take place within, or between, organisations, provided the financial systems work properly and allow properly constructed contracts to be set.

The guidance[8] issued to the NHS on the change from old-style contracts to Long-Term Service Agreements[9] states the Agreements should be client/service-based, rather than based on institutions, and that they 'will be dynamic, incorporating incentives for improving quality and cost effectiveness' (p 12).

How all this will be done in practice remains to be seen. Leaving aside the practicalities, the separation of contracts from provision opens the way for modifying the boundaries of existing formal organisations so as to reflect the way that services are actually delivered. A study[10] by Newchurch makes a similar point:

> *The accepted boundaries of the acute general hospital are largely a matter of convention and convenience. Many of the arguments for linkage between clinical services and specialties are declining, the case for co-location being primarily economic, focusing on the cost of facilities and support service. Hospitals are not homogeneous organisations but more heterogeneous, with services tending to have stronger links along the pathway of patient care, rather than across specialties. Increasing specialisation and sub-specialisation, coupled with the distributed technology, may mean that patients and carers increasingly identify with particular service organisations, focused on specific ailments, interventions or body-systems, rather than an amorphous hospital.* (p 6)

In other words, the connections between hospital and community may be stronger than the connections between parts of hospitals – apart from the basic infrastructure and support services.

Already the effective boundaries of the hospital have been shifting as a result of changes in control over facilities. As noted in Chapter Five, the area of consultation and diagnosis within hospitals has become an area of boundary shift, in respect of control rather than in physical terms. Open-access clinics, direct booking of tests and appointments and direct access to the results of tests effectively put these hospital facilities within the control of GPs without any shift in formal responsibility for the provision of the services concerned.

However, the shift in purchasing power, initially through total purchasing and now through primary care groups, has probably been decisive in many cases in encouraging such shifts. In the case of emergency admissions, for example, some total purchasers[11] developed control and monitoring systems that allowed them to monitor the progress of their patients through hospitals. In effect, this meant that the way the hospitals were used and the extent they were used were determined externally to the hospital itself.

These examples indicate that the boundary between hospital and community or specialist and generalist can vary, if the contractual structure allows it, on an incremental basis. However, the Newchurch arguments, already reflected in Chapters Three and Four, suggest that there might be grounds for a more radical change in the way the boundary is defined.

Following the arguments set out in Chapters Four and Five, systems of care for children and others that run across all providers could be contractually integrated, with the management of the programme allocated to one provider or another. The partnership arrangements provided for under the 1999 Health Act envisage a range of possibilities for combining services, including the use of providers as contract holders. This opens the way for systems of care to be defined, commissioned and managed across the boundaries of health and social care. Argument over whether geriatrics and paediatrics are community or hospital specialties would be beside the point.

As far as the hospital is concerned, the result is the so-called 'airport model', with the systems of care representing the airlines using the hospital facilities after contractual negotiation, and passengers flowing freely between them. This model recasts the internal conflicts of the hospital as a single formal organisation into a series of external negotiations (which might become conflictual) about access to hospital services.

The same issues would have to be addressed within community-based services. The national service frameworks and the proposals for managed clinical networks both identify roles for general practice and other community professionals. But within the UK the nature of the GP role means it is virtually impossible to make such links.[12] It would be possible, however, if some degree of specialisation within general medical services was formally recognised along the lines discussed in Chapter Four and if those adopting this role came to be employed by community or primary care trusts. This would open the way for community-based specialists of any discipline to be part of a 'virtual' organisation, which served a particular disease or client group, and which comprised contributions from all relevant providers. The degree of 'virtuality' would be reduced by the 'reality' of flows of finance through contracts, particularly if those contracts embodied performance standards and targets and possible sanctions for poor performance.

Organisational integration

The 'hard' barriers arising at the boundaries of formal organisations have long been seen as one of the obstacles to the effective working of the NHS. If we were still conducting our thought experiment, therefore, we might wish to assume that the NHS was in fact a single organisation so that this form of boundary did not matter.

That would still leave other organisational boundaries to traverse, such as those with social care providers, not to mention the vast range of organisations whose responsibilities bear on the prevention of ill health. But even if organisational integration were achieved within health care itself, the sheer size of the resulting organisation would bring with it difficulties of its own. Moreover, as the evidence referred to in Chapter Two indicates, organisational integration does not guarantee clinical integration – if it did, the care pathways now being slowly developed within hospitals would have been defined already.

The evidence cited in Chapter Three and the experience of hospital re-engineering[13] have served to underline the repeated and apparently endemic failure of formal management structures to ensure that patient pathways work. In practice, the formal hierarchies of control do not work, i.e. they neither avoid conflict nor reliably succeed in achieving the effective integration of the contribution of the various parts of the hospital. Similarly, in Northern Ireland, the formal integration of health and social care provision has achieved little.[14] In what follows, therefore, we do not pursue the question of whether unification across all contributing care providers would be beneficial.[15] Instead, we turn next to considering the case for organisational separation for some care providers.

Organisational separation

The case for separation is most easily made where, as with care for eyes and teeth, the services suit small-scale local delivery and where the clinical connections between these and other services are limited. Both these care systems, though largely provided by the private sector, operate, insofar as they supply services to NHS patients, within rules that tightly define which procedures form part of the NHS and which do not, and what can be charged for. These rules act in lieu of the gatekeeping role of the GP, controlling both what patients can get and what professionals can provide within the scope of the NHS. Furthermore, as noted in Chapter Six, users can generally be relied upon to choose the right entry point.

These services have had a history of separation from the rest of the NHS, going back to its origins.[16] Mental health provides an instructive contrast. The mental health service has been through two main transformations: first, a merger with general hospital services and then a shift in the balance between hospital and community in favour of the latter. Now the typical form of organisation at local level is a separate trust or a division of a community trust.

The case for this switch rests in part on the importance of the links between health and other services that have to be made at local level and, in part, on changing views as to the nature of the service. From the early 1970s onwards, the emphasis in mental health policy switched away from institutional treatment[17] towards ensuring that users of the service are linked in effectively to housing and employment as well as other mainstream services, all of which will inevitably remain organisationally distinct. The links with the main hospital service within a district general hospital, which the 1962 Hospital Plan endorsed and which came to replace the old style isolated mental hospitals, came to be seen as less important, though this form of provision continued in many areas.[18]

In principle, GPs remain the access controllers. But, as noted in Chapter Four, many users make contact with the Service directly and referral to specialists is often exercised either by community nurses or professionals in other services. For this reason, it can be argued that the process of separation should go further, following the arguments set out above for community-based specialists.

A different case for separation may be made for services that, by virtue of their specialisation and the rarity of the conditions they deal with, serve very large catchment areas. Such a case has been put forward for the continuation of the so-called 'specialist trusts' formed as a result of the 1991 reforms. Proponents of this form of trust argued,[19] using the Royal National Orthopaedic Trust as an example, that:

> ... *being part of an organisation which deals with neuro-musculos-skeletal problems rather than being part of a multi-disciplinary organisation allowed a highly focused vision which makes for increased efficiency*. (p 17)

The notion of the hospital as 'focused factory' has been put forward for other functions and has, in part, been proposed with the NHS National Plan for elective care and diagnostics centres that 'will separate routine hospital surgery from hospital emergency work so they can concentrate on getting waiting times down' (para 4.8). The implicit assumption is that such a focus cannot be achieved within existing hospital trusts through managerial devolution.[20]

A similar proposal has been made for emergency care. The report[21] cited in Chapter Five put forward two models for emergency care, the first based on collaboration – essentially a continuation of current practice – and the second based on a single organisation:

> *All the resources to deliver emergency care, from first point of contact to definitive care, would be managed within a single organisation. The delivery of elective or planned care would be separately organised, structured and resourced. Within one system emergency care would be delivered up to the point of definitive diagnosis and/or appropriate management plan, resulting in the safe discharge of patients to self-care, specialist medical or surgical care or community-based chronic disease care.*
>
> *This model could include within one organisation all the routes of access to emergency care (including NHS Direct and the ambulance service) as well as the primary care, community care, mental health and acute secondary care components to emergency care*. (p 12)

The report does not set out to attempt to determine what the advantages of this approach over the collaborative model might be nor how the contractual interfaces within the hospital would be negotiated. But the general arguments set out in Chapter Three in favour of systems of care would form the basis of the case for organisational separation, together with the need to exercise greater control over access, as discussed in Chapter Six.

The case for giving emergency care organisational separation is arguably greater than for other care systems based on disease or client group, because 'time is brain' (page 96) and hence the need for the effective linking of all the service elements contributing to the system all the greater. It would also underpin the case for emergency medical care within hospitals becoming a specialty in its own right.[22] The same logic could apply to any system of care, either in the form of clinician co-operatives or care system trusts, for which at present the NHS does not provide. We consider these in the next section.

The value of formal provider organisations

We have argued that it is useful to make a basic distinction between systems of care defined by reference to patient groups, and services defined by reference to providers. In practice, it is the latter that have provided the basis for formal organisations rather than the former. But this may not be inevitable.

Within the NHS, as a publicly financed system, the need for a formal organisational structure has been self-evident. But the justification for particular organisational forms is less clear. With the 1990 NHS and Community Care Act, however, a new form of organisation – the trust – was introduced in the expectation that it would lead to specific benefits.

The argument for trusts put forward in the Working Paper[23] were:

- a stronger sense of local ownership and pride
- encouragement of local initiative
- an increase in choice
- greater competition
- improved quality of service
- increased efficiency.

Against the background of this analysis, most of the features claimed for the new form of organisation seem irrelevant. They do not bear on the central weakness in service delivery with which we began, in particular how to ensure that the elements required for patient care pathways are in the right place at the right time. The question, therefore, is: what is the role of a formal organisation, not based on a system of care, within a health care delivery system consisting of a series of interlocking systems of care?

One answer is that formal organisation is required for all those elements that contribute to systems of care but which are not exclusively within any one. This is the central argument for the hospital as the focus for a formal organisation, since hospitals are the main sites for both the human and the physical resources that several care systems make use of. The hospital could be said to act as co-ordinator of claims for new facilities where joint investment decisions[24] have to be made and as arbiter between different claims for the use of joint facilities on a day-to-day basis.

A related argument is that boundaries between care systems should not be fixed and that it is easier to move them *within* one formal organisation rather than *between* formal organisations. In practice, both are difficult. In the early 1990s, the shift from hospital to community was often thwarted in part by the formal boundary but also in part from informal professional pressures. In principle, the answer lies in more informed and powerful purchasers, but in practice informed purchasing leading to service change proved to be rare.[25] Neither hierarchies nor contracts have turned out to be effective instruments of control.

Another possible role for formal organisation is that of a policing device for care systems. The introduction of the notion of clinical governance with responsibility focused on chief executives and boards suggests this interpretation. But these arrangements do not reflect the realities of how hospitals work now, still less how they will do so, if national service frameworks and other care systems are fully implemented within which clinicians have responsibilities to colleagues in other organisations and the standards of care to be aimed at are set nationally. Furthermore, it is at odds with the notion that national service frameworks and clinical networks should have management systems of their own.

Thus, none of these answers is entirely convincing. Is there an alternative? The logic of an approach to health care delivery based on systems of care is that these should be the prime unit for accountability and hence have some degree of both organisational and financial independence – in effect, becoming trusts in their own right.

This will appear a fantastical notion to those professionals who potentially may contribute to several. The notion of dual (triple?) lines of accountability is familiar but nonetheless hard to get right in practice, particularly so if the demands along each line become more explicit and precise. But this dilemma has to be faced if pathways and systems of care are to be the basis for care delivery.[26] So far, however, it has been ignored, or more accurately, acknowledged but not seen as requiring institutional change.[27]

Conclusion

We concluded in Chapter Four that systems of care were likely to be interlocking rather than distinct entities each with their own staff and assets. It follows from this that systems of care and organisational structures can never be perfectly aligned. The task of finding the best overall structure for a health care system necessarily involves a series of compromises between different forms of integration.

If pathways are to be clearly defined and the potential advantages of systems of care realised, then clinical integration of the kind envisaged in Box 7.1 must exist. But the further clinical integration proceeds away from informal co-operation based on long-standing custom and practice and towards formal co-operation based on precisely defined procedures, the more the question will arise as to how the boundaries between systems of care relate to formal organisation.

Because of supply side links, the removal of organisational barriers in one place will lead to others appearing elsewhere.[28] A system of care for the elderly or for children, formally organised across the current boundary of hospital and community, would create a new organisational boundary within both. The gains from the development of one system of care may be at the expense of costs arising where patients or professionals straddle the new boundary.

In this respect, the health care delivery system is no different to the large business corporation that has to decide whether to structure by geography, product or function, whether to focus on one core function, and whether to buy in the other services it needs. The 'right' answers to these issues appear to be in a constant state of flux as different management fads rule. In the case of the NHS, the current fad has been for horizontal mergers between hospital trusts or between community trusts in the hope[29] that management costs would be saved. At the same time, however, the opposite approach has been adopted for the provision of capital assets, where the private finance initiative rests on the assumption that separation of key functions will give rise to greater efficiency.[30] Both may be right, but in neither case has the Government set out in any detail precisely why contracts are better for hospital assets and organisational integration is better for (some) health care services. But that question – which boundaries are best defined in terms of formal organisation and which by contracts? – is the central structural issue for the organisation of health care delivery.

References

1. Although attempts have been and continue to be made to 'regulate' referral patterns, they remain persistently 'unregulated'. The National Institute of Clinical Excellence has begun to attempt to impose some 'order' through the issue of referral guidelines.
2. In principle, the introduction of the electronic patient record and development of information systems will make this process easier.
3. The work of the Intensive Care National Audit and Research Centre and other similar networks fall into this category. The exchange and sharing is essentially of information only: the sharing allows larger samples to be built up quickly, benchmarking of performance to be put on a proper basis, and so on.
4. Standing Medical Advisory Committee, 1997.
5. Scottish Office, 1998.
6. Scottish Office, 1999.
7. As an unpublished paper by the London Region makes clear, a clinical network will involve a large number of other collective activities, including data analysis, provision of information to patients, research, training, quality assurance, development of protocols and modification, and improvement of patient pathways.
8. Department of Health, 1998a.
9. The logic for this change was set out in *The New NHS* (Secretary of State for Health, 1997).
10. Newchurch, 1999.
11. Mays *et al.*, 1998.
12. It would imply the GP contract being disaggregated into a series of contracts for each system of care.
13. Packwood *et al.*, 1992.
14. This point was acknowledged in a recent official report on the management of winter pressures in Northern Ireland (Department of Health Social Services and Public Safety, 2000, see para 5.16).
15. See Robinson and Casalino, 1996, for a discussion of this and related issues.
16. Hill and Woodcock, 1949.
17. Peck and Parker, 1998.
18. The author was told when carrying out research for Harrison and Prentice, 1996, that the links with A&E were more important than community links (e.g. in cases of self-harm), and hence mental health should be part of the hospital service.

19. NHS Trust Federation, 1997.
20. The experience of attempts to create elective care centres in Wales tends to support this view (see House of Commons, 1997).
21. Coffey and Mythen, 2000.
22. The New Health Network report sets out a series of next steps for emergency services that includes the development of new systems of emergency care and their evaluation. By implication it argues that these are prior steps to any organisational change.
23. Department of Health, 1989.
24. As noted above, some proponents of managed clinical networks assume they will have responsibility for investment decisions. Some assets will be specific to each network, but others will be shared with other systems of care.
25. See, for example, Audit Commission, 1996a and 1997a.
26. The same issues have arisen in a very different health care system. In the US, the term 'carve outs' has come to be used for specialist and organisationally separate providers (see, for example, Pristave *et al.*, 1995, and Kurowski, 1997). The debate continues on their merits and the range of services this form of organisation might be suitable for. See also Robinson, 1999. More than any other writer, Robinson has monitored changes in the US health care system from the 'hierarchies and contracts' angle.
27. The NHS Cancer Plan (NHS Executive, 2000c), for example, proposes that chief executives of trusts involved in a local cancer system should combine to create a line of accountability.
28. Leutz, 1998, compares British and American attempts to integrate services. One of his 'Laws of Integration' runs 'your integration is my fragmentation'.
29. As McClenahan and Mumford, 1999, have pointed out, the evidence from outside the health sector points the other way.
30. For a wider discussion of the private finance initiative, see Boyle and Harrison, 2000a and 2000b.

Chapter Eight

Systems of care and the knowledge base

We have argued elsewhere[1] that, at least as far as the NHS is concerned, the search for knowledge has been primarily focused on episodes of treatment rather than the health care delivery systems within which treatment takes place. This bias reflects two main factors:

- the bias in professional culture towards the clinical encounter with the patient rather than system design
- the large role that private sector research plays in determining how health care systems operate. The vast majority of this effort is also focused on the specific intervention, usually a drug but sometimes a procedure, rather than the broader context in which the intervention is provided.

These two factors share a common intellectual culture that sees progress in health care as depending on the development of new forms of treatment and which assumes that the search for these should be conducted by methods that rely for their success, like any scientific endeavour, on the isolation of the impact of individual elements through appropriate very carefully defined experimental procedures.

In contrast, the development of systems emphasises different elements of care delivery:

- the routing of patients to specific care systems
- the interdependence of different parts of a care system
- the interdependence between care systems
- the boundaries of care systems and their match with patient needs, particularly where there is multiple morbidity
- the role of users in determining how effectively care systems operate
- the links between professions, training, and the definition of care systems
- the impact of the institutional context on the way in which care systems operate.

None of these is a new theme and we have been able to draw on research findings that bear on all of them. But our analysis has also revealed that much of the evidence bearing on what are the central issues within the design of care systems is ambiguous or partial. And, with respect to some of the issues raised, there is very little evidence indeed. As Fisher and Welch[2,3] point out in their discussion of the unintended consequences of medical care: 'We are missing a level of analysis, the system' (p 452).

The weakness of the current situation is well illustrated through the national service frameworks. These aim to be evidence-based, but our earlier analysis of Calman/Hine[4] revealed weaknesses in the evidence and analysis relating to:

- the proposed cancer care system itself
- the links between it and other systems
- links with non-clinical areas such as finance.

These gaps meant that, although the Committee's proposals were plausible, they were not convincing, certainly not to the standards of evidence that clinicians working within the field would seek to apply to their own interventions.

The subsequent national service frameworks for mental health and coronary heart disease have recognised that their proper implementation requires much more knowledge and information than was available at the time they were drawn up. The first part of this chapter considers these requirements in more detail. The second considers the policy implications.

System description

The way of analysing health care systems set out in Chapters Three and Four implies a radical change to the way in which any one whole delivery system, such as the NHS, or any one part of it, such as cancer care, is described. At the most basic level this means that provider-based statistics must be replaced with data based on patients' flows from the beginning to the end of their pathways. This information is required not only to provide accounts of how many patients get treated and where, but also to provide the basis for monitoring and improving the performance of each system of care.

The introduction of care pathways for narrowly defined groups of users impacts not only on the recording of the flows along the pathway and the events along the way, but also on the use of such information to provide the basis quality monitoring and a continuous process of improvement. In other words, the audit process falls directly out of the routine collection and management of the data describing the progress of patients.[5]

There are no data of this kind for any user group that might be used to describe the flows of patients through any care system, however defined. The national service frameworks for mental health and coronary heart disease and the NHS Cancer Plan do not even attempt to map out these flows. Similarly, there has been no attempt at such a mapping for either emergency care or elective care despite the major policy interest in both of these. The report of the National Beds Inquiry, despite its focus on care for the elderly, did not attempt to map the pathways through which elderly people gain access to hospital nor the routes they take after leaving it, still less the numbers using any of these pathways. As the Audit Commission in its report on diabetes[6] points out, without such a basis, little can be said about whether local or national systems of care are being effective at addressing the needs of the population as a whole. In some parts of the country, however, registers of people suffering from particular conditions exist or have existed (see Box 8.1).

At national/regional level, the only condition systematically recorded is cancer but, as the Select Committee on Science and Technology has noted,[7] the organisation and funding of cancer registries are on a haphazard footing, and their very existence 'the result of historical accident rather than strategic planning' (para 98).

Box 8.1 A local CHD register

The register has been developed locally and can be changed to respond to the needs of the service and current developments.

Key features include:
accurate data which can be used to audit the service provided by the trust;
increasing coverage of the register in primary care for audit purposes;
the use of a standard form for collecting clinical information which has improved record-keeping and helps with continuity of care;
a perception of increasing accuracy of primary care based data and wider 'ownership' of data; and
stronger links with primary care through visits by the specialist diabetes nurse which has helped to strengthen continued professional development as well as improve record-keeping

Source: Audit Commission, 2000a.

The registries do not, however, record the information vital to describing how the care system works, i.e. the times and experience of patients moving through it even though they do provide an essential underpinning of any attempt to understand mortality trends.[8,9]

While patient flows and their care and outcome experience clearly must provide the centrepiece of any system description, the care system approach also has major implications for the description of providers. Workforce and financial information must be available on the same basis, to provide the means for estimating the cost of each system and the implications for financial and workforce planning of developing the system. No such data are available now, as a recent study[10] of cancer care found:

> *Detailed information needed to plan and manage individual patients' treatment is fragmented and disconnected. Different specialties and even more, different organisations, collect similar information in different ways, using different definitions, format and content even of similar data items, and different computer systems or paper-only records. Notes of different professions are often filed separately, inaccessible to other members of the clinical team.*

The national service frameworks acknowledge this. In the case of coronary heart disease,[11] the framework states that:

> *Development of a CHD Information Strategy will start during the latter half of 1999/2000 to specify the practical and cost-effective steps to support the information requirements of this NSF. This will include consideration of a Healthcare Framework ... and its application in different data environments. This Healthcare Framework will provide an integrating mechanism for viewing needs, interventions, and performance indicators together. It will also be a vehicle for comparative analysis based on national standard groupings of data.* (para 5.55, p 103)

The framework goes on to indicate that the electronic patient record will make this easier:

> *4.19 The Information for Health Strategy anticipates that data will be held in electronic patient records coded in clinical terms, and structured in a way that allows access to relevant parts of the record. Electronic messages will be defined to ensure accurate transmission and receipt of information. This structure and consistency of information will allow extraction of data and analysis for several*

> *purposes. In particular it will support audit of the process and outcome of care and much of the information required for the indicators in the NHS Performance Assessment Framework will be collectable in this way. The electronic record will therefore provide the source of detailed clinical information to monitor how well services are delivered.* (NSF, CHD, p 78)

Although the Government is pressing on with the development of the electronic patient record, there are a number of obstacles to its rapid introduction, such as concern about access to records and confidentiality, as well as delays in actually introducing the relevant computing systems. But, as the national service framework goes on to acknowledge, a great deal of work remains to be done, even if the electronic records do become available:

> *4.21 Another major task will be the resolution of the practical difficulties in extracting and using the information. Although the information may be held in electronic format, it may be difficult to extract the relevant data items and analyse them consistently. Many units do not yet have the necessary skills or resources to exploit the information potentially available to them, and even if they do, they cannot be sure that they are extracting and analysing data consistently with other units. To enable local units to have comparable benchmarking information, and for the NHS Executive to have reliable monitoring information, a nationally agreed way of extracting and analysing data from electronic patient records is required.* (NSF, CHD, p 78)

As this extract makes clear, the process of getting information on this system of care has scarcely begun.

In 1998, the first set of so-called 'reference costs'[12] for hospitals were published, the first step towards introducing some degree of transparency into NHS costs.[13] But these focused on specific hospital procedures, not the costs associated with the flow of patients through the hospital as a whole. For the reasons set out in Chapter Three, the right 'costing unit' is the patient pathway, i.e. a linked series of episodes. But the ability to do the costing on this basis does not yet exist, either within hospitals or between hospitals and other parts of the health care system.

System behaviour

The ability to describe a flow of patients, their clinical experience and their associated costs along a set of care pathways is, however, just the beginning of understanding how systems of care work. We argued in Chapters Four and Six that the notion of a system of health care delivery comprised not only care facilities and processes but also the behaviour of the individuals working in it and those using it. We have argued in Chapters Three and Six that the level of demand experienced by the health care delivery system is in part dependent on the way that the system is itself configured, both in physical terms and also in terms of the rules of access that apply. The same is true within the system itself, i.e. the rules of access of, for example, community professionals to hospital resources will determine to some degree the extent to which they are used, particularly if use implies payment.

As far as the professional is concerned, the association of protocols and other decision rules with pathways, disease management and so on, can be seen as attempts to limit the extent to which professional behaviour can vary and hence the need to understand and predict it. However, as Haycox and his colleagues[14] have argued, these pose 'system' issues of their own because of their ramifications. Hence, they conclude that: 'The only secure basis for guidelines is a comprehensive assessment of all consequences (direct and indirect) of a new treatment' (p 393). In other words, the way in which professionals as individuals or as parts of organisations respond to intervention designed to 'manage' their behaviour requires understanding in its own right.[15]

Furthermore, however successful the introduction of guidelines proves to be, in many of the areas where care systems fail the reasons stem from unpredictable events and from interfaces between systems where other factors come into play – where, for example, financial rules influence the way routing or other choices are made. A study[16] of safety in health care systems found:

> *The enormous complexity of health care is a daunting obstacle to those trying to study safety systematically. Everything, it seems, is connected to everything else, and every thread of action and cause is wound into a great Gordian knot.*

The study suggested that one way cutting through the knot is to focus on gaps rather than 'whole systems':

> *Gaps themselves mark the areas of vulnerability and show the mechanism by which complexity flows through health care to individual patients. Pursuing gaps is a method that allows technical work to guide both research into and improvement in safety.* (p 794)

The behaviour of users as they pass through a hospital care pathway has little scope for variation and does not appear to require 'explanation' or explicit understanding. But once we stand back and view the wider perspective of the elective care system as a whole, the arguments set out in Chapter Four suggest that users can exercise considerable choice.[17] The same is true of urgent care, particularly where users have a number of access points. Indeed, for all care systems, particularly those such as cancer, where delay may be important, the decision to access the service at the point of first contact – either GP or screening – may be vital to a successful outcome.

The task of understanding user behaviour is most critical for the emergency care system, since this is the most user-driven part of the health care delivery system, and the one with the least effective system of entry control in place. The amount of work carried out into forecasting use and admissions at hospital level as well as community services remains small, and what has been done serves to point up the complexities of the task. Nearly all studies of the rise of emergency admissions in recent years have come to the conclusion that many factors are at work, most of which are not readily quantifiable[18] with existing data sets.

Furthermore, as we have argued above, the way in which users behave both outside the formal system and as they approach it is equally important for determining how effective systems of care are relative to measures taken outside, including both the provision of information and advice to potential users, and wider measures directed at the health of the public at large.[19]

The NHS R&D programme has recognised the need to consult users on research priorities but has yet to focus on understanding the interactions between users and services. Yet, as argued in Chapter Six, this is an essential element of the demand management task. In the case of NHS Direct, an evaluation of the pilot sites relied upon statements of intention rather than actual behaviour. The alternative – tracking actual behaviour – would have been much more difficult and much more expensive.[20]

But if any system of care is to be properly managed, it will require the development of new and more ambitious approaches to the evaluation of the impact of service innovation, e.g. through the use of survey techniques commonly used in transport planning, which involve intensive and expensive recording of what travellers actually do. The National Patient Surveys[21] represent a useful start, but they do not collect detailed information about 'care journeys' – the health equivalent of what people experience when they use transport services.[22]

System design

The national service frameworks embody a clear intention to use and develop indicators to monitor progress in their implementation. While this is clearly an important task, it does not bear on the central question of how to get the best overall system design. The mental model implicit in the frameworks, as well as in the NHS Cancer Plan, is that they should define what is best at each stage of the care pathway, rather than attempting to define the best combination of interventions taking the care system as a whole.

There is now a vast literature on the evaluation of health care services. However, this is almost entirely focused, like much of the clinical literature, on specific interventions rather than alternative configurations of health care delivery systems. As numerous texts acknowledge, care pathways and similar developments have not been subject to rigorous evaluation. Once the focus moves to the broader canvas of a system of care, then the task of determining which is the best combination of interventions or what contribution the separate elements of a series of interventions makes to the overall process is much more difficult. In the case of hospitals, for example, interpretation of the evidence, which, to a varying degree supports the case for concentrating certain activities in fewer hospitals, is difficult, precisely because a large number of factors other than size of hospital or number of operations per surgeon are involved, as well as patient-related confounding factors.

To take one example, a study[23] of the performance of A&E departments in England found that the general trend has been favourable, i.e. more lives were being saved than several years ago after allowing for changes in the severity of those seeking treatment. But the reasons for the improvement were not apparent, even though the study drew on a very detailed and extensive data set, much better than is available for the parts of most other care systems. The authors were led to conclude that the improvement might be attributable to the changes in staffing that had been introduced to improve performance, but the study itself could not demonstrate this. Given the limited number of departments and the large number of potential factors, these reasons might be impossible to identify with confidence, even though the study was able to standardise for changes in the nature of the conditions treated.

The larger the care system, the greater the challenge. A study of stroke care[24] found that the evidence confirmed that dedicated stroke units did perform better than other ways of providing for stroke victims, but the available data did not allow the contribution of their various elements to be estimated:

> *In this systematic review we have identified randomised trials comparing two broad and ill defined systems of care: a stroke unit 'black box' and a conventional care 'black box'. This initial comparison has allowed us to conclude that improvements in the organisation of inpatient stroke care can bring about important improvements in the recovery of patients. However, although these are important conclusions they only represent a first step towards delivering better stroke care. These simple conclusions conceal the underlying diversity and complexity of the individual trials and the systems of care which they were comparing. As this review is essentially a pragmatic exercise to identify reliable information to guide the care of individual stroke patients, we must explore the diversity within the individual trials. However, there is a paradox: by asking increasingly more specific questions by carrying out 'subgroup analyses', we are likely to produce more statistically unreliable answers.* (pp 49–50)

A similar conclusion was reached with respect to maternity care in the community:[25]

> *No two schemes are quite the same ... Even when two schemes appear similar on paper, the personalities behind the projects, the nature of the population served, the size of the workload and many other features will vary, and these are likely to be major determinants of success or failure. Given the large number of parameters involved, we must be very careful in reaching conclusions about the causes of different outcomes.* (p 131)

In these cases, fine tuning around the black box solution may be appropriate: different providers can adapt different variations. But it may well be that all the options cannot be tested in combination as there would be too many of them.[26] The only route, therefore, may be system simulation, which in principle allows different policies to be 'tried out' in combination without actually implementing them. But this is only a partial solution, as we note below.

Finally, there are structural features that are so central to the overall system that they become almost unresearchable. One example is the role of the gatekeeper and the structural divide between community and hospital-based clinicians. Research can and has been done on small changes in role. There is, for example, a large body of work around the issues of open access to, and GP control of hospital resources such as diagnostics, which allow GPs (and others) direct referral routes to human resources such as physiotherapy, as well as other shifts of responsibilities such as may occur within shared care schemes.[27] But major shifts in role cannot be tackled in this way since they imply too many changes to evaluate by careful controlled experiment.

One option for evaluating major changes is to compare the performance of different health care delivery systems. As noted in Chapter Five, there have been a number of attempts to do so based on cross-country comparisons. Starfield,[28] for example, found that the existence of universal primary care was correlated with both good health outcomes and user satisfaction, and there has also been work on the balance, at national level, between specialists and generalists.

Such results, however, cannot identify the elements of generalist care that produce the outcomes identified. In cases such as these, the only route may be experiment at the micro level. The experimental relaxation of the regulatory framework provided for by the 1997 Primary Care Act opened the way for change by providing evidence of the viability of alternative delivery mechanisms, such as the open access schemes referred to above. However, by their nature, experiments of this kind, however well evaluated, shed no light on the value of the change if other aspects of the care pathway were changed at the same time. In the case of emergency admissions, for example, some total purchasing pilots[29] tested the value of using community-based nurses within the hospital to check on the progress of patients referred by the participating practices. This appeared beneficial, but the same result might not be obtained if hospitals themselves improved their bed management and discharge policies.

The difficulties of attribution, however, are all the greater when other forms of intervention, primarily those of a preventive nature, are taken into account. In the case of cancer, screening programmes for breast and cervical cancer have been in place in the UK for about ten years. But some recent assessments of screening programmes[30] have suggested that they do not confer benefits, partly because screening imposes health costs itself and partly because the advantages of a formally organised programme are much lower than previously thought, perhaps because in the countries surveyed women were ready to present themselves anyway. As a consequence, the advantages of the systematic call and recall procedures of the programmes were reduced.

Experiments are harder to devise and implement where they require change from a number of agencies. In the case of the 'research experiment' at the Trauma Centre at Stoke,[31] for example, the impact was limited by the failure to change ambulance operations – not the responsibility of the hospital trust hosting the Centre – and referral practices in neighbouring hospitals, which meant that the Centre was not receiving all the patients who would have benefited from it. This suggests that there is a central role for the identification, implementation and monitoring of a small number of major experiments – a point to which we return below.

Perhaps a more serious problem is the definition of what is in and what is out of the system of care being evaluated. There is a long-standing debate about the contribution of clinical care to the observed increases in life expectancy[32] arising from McKeown's suggestion that the bulk of the improvement in life expectancy in the last century was due to public health and other policies rather than improvements in health care. This debate remains unresolved.[33]

Essentially the same issues arise with the health care interventions that a health care delivery system comprises. In the case of the national service frameworks currently being developed, no attempt has been made to estimate the expected contribution of changes within the wider environment or in personal behaviour to the hoped-for gains in mortality from these conditions. Instead, a range of preventive measures is set out, without any indication of their relative importance or the nature and extent of the interaction between them and the outcome of care.[34]

One way forward would be to establish and monitor different care systems in different parts of the country. There would be ethical difficulties with that (even though there is extensive variation is the current situation[35]), but even if it were done, major difficulties would remain, particularly changes during the monitoring period in the availability of drugs or other interventions, as well as changes in the wider environment.

These points might suggest that systems of care can never be properly evaluated or their design optimised, even in the absence of technical change in treatment modes. However, even the availability of a simple description of how each care system works would stand some chance of reducing the risk of double-counting benefits from interventions working in series, as in a programme for cancer care. Such a description could, for example, establish whether changes in presentation were occurring or whether, given a set of people with similar personal and disease characteristics, treatment had become more effective.

Simulation models

The absence of basis data, the complexity of system evaluation and the costs of dealing with both, might suggest that there is little chance, either analytically or in practice, of designing, implementing and modifying systems of care on the basis of a substantive understanding of how well they work. One way forward is simulation.

Simulation is now, and has been for some time, routine in aviation and other industries both for design and training. Within the health field, it has been slow to have an impact. Although the potential of computer-based models was recognised in the late 1960s, interest evaporated. There are some more recent examples of service models largely focused on specific functions such as A&E and ICUs and hospital beds.[36]

A central difficulty in the health field, in contrast to aviation and other industrial fields, is that the basis for projecting outside current experience is much weaker – there is no parallel to the understanding of the behaviour of aircraft, subject to external forces, that allows simulators to mimic accurately real world aerodynamic behaviour. Nevertheless, simulation in health care, once it is focused on a whole system of care, has a range of uses:

- It is of heuristic value, i.e. as a source of insights and a stimulus to the imagination, to suggest areas where experiments may be beneficial or where difficulties may arise if specific changes are made. At the level of the care pathway, however, where detailed data can be collected, the accuracy of a model of the flow process may be systematically checked.
- It can provide a means of integrating knowledge based on partial studies, for example hip fracture.[37]
- It can explore different means of delivering care, including variations around an established model, at relatively low cost.
- It can identify research possibilities and gaps in basic information.[38]

So far, however, the NHS has shown itself reluctant to invest sufficient resources to realise these benefits.

System-wide comparisons

As we have noted already, it is impossible within the confines of one national health care delivery system to evaluate some of its central features. Ironically, the closer the system comes to uniformity through the development of national services frameworks, the greater that difficulty will be.

As noted already, one way forward is international comparisons. But progress will be slow: the data gaps described above for the UK, but not exclusive to it, bedevil cross-national work. In the case of cancer care, for example, cross-national estimates of performance published by the Cancer Research Campaign[39] failed, because of data gaps, to allow for disease stage at presentation. Furthermore, the proportion of patients covered by the respective national studies varied a great deal – in some countries it was around 1 per cent, whereas about 50 per cent of the UK is covered, giving rise to the possibility that well-organised systems were represented in only some countries and were not the general experience.

Nevertheless, even a simple description of how different systems of care work may be illuminating. For example, emergency care within community and hospitals is organised very differently in different countries, but no authoritative comparisons are available, as compared to the very detailed comparisons of finance and institutional arrangements at national level.[40]

Restructuring research commissioning

We argued in Chapter Five that the thought experiment with which we began required the training of professionals to be geared to services defined independently of those professions. The same applies to the generation of the knowledge base that those professionals embody and make use of. These points may seem self-evident, but even if we take the R&D supported from public funds through the Department of Health and the NHS, the notion that the production of knowledge should be closely linked to service delivery is relatively new.

The first major attempt to link research to service needs began in 1991 following a report from the House of Lords.[41] That report identified a nearly universal failure to link research to the 'needs of the Service'. Accepting the general drift of the report, the Government established what was then called an 'R&D initiative' under the direction of Michael Peckham, and he in turn published *Research for Health*.[42] That led to the development of a series of new research programmes combined with the introduction of a new way of allocating money for research. Following the Culyer report[43] on the way that research was being funded within the NHS, an attempt has been made to shift research work away from the teaching hospital to other locations.

With the possible exception of a programme covering the primary–secondary interface, the resulting research has been largely traditional in terms of subject and method, that is to say focused on small parts of the overall system. The Interface programme, although focused on a structural issue, resulted in a series of apparently unrelated projects and no synthesis of the results, in part because no provision was made for this and in part because the programme was not founded on a clear view of the context into which the results should fit. In other words, the 'needs of the Service' continued to be defined in traditional terms.

In March 2000, however, a programme focused on Organisation and Delivery was launched. Its prospectus[44] set out the following priorities:

- *Organising health services around the needs of the patient.*
- *User involvement.*
- *Continuity of care.*
- *Co-ordination/integration across organisations.*
- *Inter-professional working.*
- *Workforce issues.*
- *Relationship between organisational form, function and outcomes.*
- *Implications of the communication revolution.*
- *The use of resources, such as ways of disinvesting in services and managing demand.*
- *Implementation of major national policy initiatives such as the national service frameworks for coronary heart disease and mental health.* (p 5)

This agenda does, in contrast, begin to address the system level issues. Funding for this programme remains at a very low level, however, and the programme had by the end of 2000 scarcely got off the ground.

However, the consultation paper on the commissioning of research for the NHS, issued in 2000, showed little awareness of the issues discussed here.[45] As the King's Fund argued in its response, new forms of research institution need to be devised to deal with system-wide issues cutting across traditional boundaries. Although it is obvious that they must be interdisciplinary, how exactly they should be organised remains to be worked out.[46]

Although academic research is essential, it is not the only source of relevant knowledge. The role of the auditors, particularly the Clinical Standards Advisory Group (now wound up within the Commission for Health Improvement), the National Audit Office and the Audit Commission, has vastly increased knowledge of how things work and fail, and all three have tried in studies of particular clinical conditions or broader issues to move into a systems of care framework. The Audit Commission, for example, in its study of care for elderly people,[47] set out two local health care systems configured as follows:

Table 8.1 Two local health care systems

	Area A Very long waiting lists	*Area B* No waiting lists or blocked beds
Social services position relative to SSA	Significantly above	Below
Social services gross spend on older people's services/pop. 75 plus	£1,600+	£600+
Area A also supports more people in homes and has a higher admission rate		
Social services – supported residential and nursing home placements/1000 aged 75+	54	41
Social services monthly nursing home admission rate/1000 aged 75+	1.9	0.8
Nursing home places available/ 1000 aged 75+	95	52
In Area B there are more continuing care beds, more rehabilitation beds, and the health authority has a lower readmission rate		
Health authority continuing care beds for older people/1000 aged 75+	0.8	1.8
Health authority continuing care beds for rehabilitation/1000 aged 75+	2.6	4.9
Health authority readmission rate within 90 days for people aged 75+	20%	13%
Moreover, in Area B there is more investment in the community and joint working between health and social services		
Social services intensive home care packages: per cent 6+ visits per week	26%	39%
Percentage of care packages that are multidisciplinary	3%	49%
Health authority: per cent spend on community services	8%	10%

Source: Audit Commission, 1997a, p 52.

The Audit Commission's aim in Table 8.1 was to illustrate how the various elements in this system might work in harmony – or not. However, the Commission's terms of reference and the organisational division between health and social care make it hard for them, or others, to pursue the cross-boundary system rigorously and to demonstrate the actual nature of the relationships between the various service elements.

Essentially the same is true of the Commission for Health Improvement.[48] The programme of work announced by the Commission involves visits to trusts to assess their systems of clinical management, rather than assessment of the capacity of local health economies to deal with specific issues.

Despite these weaknesses, which we return to below, the auditors represent an exceedingly valuable source of knowledge that formally organised academic research can rarely match. There is a case, therefore, for extending their capacity to carry out enquiries that are not directly linked to the audit process. Though the Audit Commission has some capacity for such work, which it exploits for national studies, this capacity is usually deployed only in support of local audits.

Conclusion

Chapter Three set out a number of reasons why focusing on systems of care could be beneficial. As this and previous chapters have shown, realising those benefits is not straightforward. The central difficulty is that the very factor that underpins the arguments for using systems of care as the basis unit for studying health care delivery makes their investigation difficult, if not impossible. The difficulties highlighted and the scale of the task even within a particular system of care may suggest accurate system description and well-found understanding of system behaviour are unreachable goals. It is, therefore, easier to identify weaknesses and gaps than to set out how the knowledge base for delivering systems of care should be strengthened. We have identified several obstacles to progress.

First, the centrepiece of the analysis running through the whole of this book is the notion of interdependence. As for service delivery, so for research and intelligence gathering; a critical question is when is it appropriate to focus on the part of a system, or supporting service, given that any change in it might impact on others. In the current state of knowledge, that question is hard to resolve. The extent and nature of interdependence, though known through experience by managers and clinicians, is rarely explored in quantitative terms – nor even systematically mapped in qualitative terms.

A second fundamental difficulty is that some system features are virtually universal – principally the main system rules. Where these are both binding and uniform, there is no scope within the system itself for isolating their impact or carrying out a fundamental assessment. Professional rules come into this category, for they too generally apply on a national basis. Experiments of the kind allowed within personal medical services under the provisions of the 1997 Act represent the first systematic approach to exploring the implications of allowing system rules to be relaxed.

Third, a focus on systems of care leads to the identification of a range of issues that stem from day-to-day interdependence. As we note in more detail below, the setting of the right financial incentives depends on knowledge of a kind that is rarely collected, e.g. the interconnections between social interventions and health outcomes, many of which are long term in nature and do not reveal themselves in the day-to-day delivery of care. In the case of Table 8.1, taken from *Coming of Age*, the links between rapid access to elective care and lower rates of emergency admissions are relatively short term, but those between higher rates of domiciliary care and admissions may not be fully apparent for years.

Fourth, the market each system serves is itself changing in ways that impinge not only on the numbers of people likely to need care but also the way in which they want to be cared for. Serious attempts to anticipate such changes, taking account of clinical, economic and social change, remain rare: the report of the National Beds Inquiry, for example, despite its 20-year time horizon, made no attempt to do this, nor has any other official paper. In large measure, these difficulties have not been confronted or even recognised, either in the national services frameworks or in the R&D programme.

As we have indicated at various points in earlier chapters, the basis for such judgements is weak. To strengthen it, there is a need to:

- Rethink R&D requirements within a systems of care framework. A start has been made to shift work in the right direction, but more needs to be done, specifically:
  - □ introducing a much greater integrative capacity: unlike the primary and secondary programme, any substantial research initiative should be accompanied by a synthesising process, using both its results and those obtainable from other sources.

- □ commissioning research around cross-cutting topics such as continuity, the first Service Delivery and Organisation programme.
- Develop design tools such as simulation, which can also be used to define research needs by focusing on critical relationships.
- Use the systems framework to define research requirements. Despite the difficulties noted, the use of the framework provided by systems of care suggests research topics that would otherwise be missed altogether or have low priority because of not being directly concerned with treatment.
- Develop cross-national studies of service delivery. At the moment, virtually the whole focus of international comparisons is on finance and the roles of private and public suppliers.

References

1. Harrison and Dixon, 2000, Chapter 11.
2. Fisher and Welch, 1999. These authors make the distinction between discrete and systemic, which is fundamental to the analysis set out here. The first is the realm of the clinician: the second is a shared realm, shared, that is, with other decision-makers.
3. Recent work on medical accidents has the same focus; see, for example, Kohn, *et al.*, 2000.
4. Harrison, 1998.
5. See, for example, Johnson, 1997.
6. Audit Commission, 2000a.
7. House of Commons, 2000.
8. The clinical information networks referred to in the previous chapter focus on hospital data.
9. The Cancer Times Waiting Audit carried out in 1998 did measure experience of waiting at all stages of the care pathway, but this was a special exercise.
10. McClenahan and Mumford, undated, mimeo unpublished.
11. Department of Health, 2000c.
12. Department of Health, 1998d.
13. The Guillebaud report recommended in the 1950s that standard costs for hospital activity should be prepared.
14. Haycox *et al.*, 1999.
15. There is a large literature on the extent to which clinicians observe protocols, but its main focus is on the impact of what the individual clinician does rather than the broader impact of the protocol on the care systems in which they work.
16. Cook *et al.*, 2000.
17. See also Harrison and New, 2000.
18. See, for example, Kendrick *et al.*, 1997. But neither this nor most other work in the field considers the individual as a decision-maker.

19. See, for example, Mulligan, 2000b.
20. Some attempts have been made at local level.
21. Airey and Erens, 1999.
22. Transport surveys may simply collect data on individual journeys, but for major plans they typically collect travel diaries for a week, along with data relating to the individuals or households involved. There has been some work done on health diaries; see Baker *et al.*, 1999.
23. Lecky *et al.*, 2000.
24. Langhorne and Dennis, 1998.
25. Marsh and Renfrew, 1999.
26. See van Weel and Knottnerus, 1999, for discussion of these issues and for suggestions as to how to deal with them.
27. See Davies, undated, Edwards *et al.*, 1996, Levy *et al.*, 1997, and Hicknan *et al.*, 1994.
28. Starfield, 1994, and Shi, 1994, 1995.
29. See Mays *et al.*, 1998.
30. Miller *et al.*, 2000.
31. Nichol *et al.*, 1995.
32. See Mulligan, 2000b, for a review of the issues.
33. A recent review by Buck *et al.*, 1999, of the techniques available for tackling this questions both current techniques and whether existing theoretical frameworks are adequate to the task.

    The complexity of the analytic problem implied by our question precludes the use of simple analytic techniques to infer a quantitative answer from the available data. Even if the requisite data were available, our discussion has cast doubt on the ability of analytic techniques to deliver convincing results ... There must be some doubt as to whether existing techniques are adequate for the task in question. (p 105)
34. The implicit model is additive, i.e. assumes that the effects of each intervention can be added to the total, with no allowance for possible interaction between them. It also takes no account of resource limits.
35. This has allowed the evaluation of alternative ways to respond to stroke; see, for example, Kalra *et al.*, 2000.
36. See, for example, Millard, 1994, 1996 and 2000, and Department of Health, 2000b.
37. Currie, 2000.
38. In the same way, a simple plotting of the care pathways in a system of care can be useful in demonstrating, for example, where the knowledge gaps are. In the case of elective care, Hamblin *et al.* attempted to locate the research evidence within the systems framework used. This showed that there were large gaps in some parts of the care system. The same result emerged from a systematic description the pathways for patients with suspected cardiac arrest. Dowie *et al.*, 1998, using a decision analysis framework (rather than simulation) that identified the number of distinct routes and routing choices faced by those responding to cardiac arrest found that there was virtually no relevant research relating to many of these choices. They

concluded that 'substantial empirical work was needed if [service] commissioning was to be even modestly evidence-based' (p 88).

39. Berino *et al.*, 1999.
40. A few small scale studies have appeared; see, for example, Sefrin and Weidringer, 1991.
41. House of Lords, 1988.
42. Department of Health, 1991.
43. Culyer, 1994.
44. NHS Executive, 2000a.
45. Department of Health, 2000f; see also King's Fund, 2000.
46. The inequalities network provides one good example. It can be accessed at: Health-Equity-Network@jiscmail.ac.uk
47. Audit Commission, 1997a.
48. The CHI site visits focus on whole institutions. However, it has recently indicated that, in association with the Audit Commission, it does intend to look at care systems, starting with cancer.

Chapter Nine

Implementing systems of care

We showed in Chapter Two that the issues with which this book is concerned have never been systematically addressed within the UK and, as a result, many have not been extensively research or analysed. Anyone attempting now to turn the thought experiment with which we began into a plan for a 'model' health care delivery system would be faced with an impossible task – impossible, that is, to carry out on the basis of a deeply considered appraisal of all the relevant options.

If the NHS, or any other established system, is to restructure its service delivery system, then in practice it would do so incrementally. And that is precisely how policy has developed through:

- national service frameworks for specific diseases and care groups
- the introduction of care pathways for some categories of care
- the development of so-called 'whole systems' to deal with winter pressures
- the introduction of financial and other measures to promote cross-boundary working, including both contracting/commissioning mechanisms and financial pooling
- the development of managed clinical networks
- the promotion of joint working in all its many guises.

While all these move the NHS in the right direction, this is in line with the analysis set out in Chapters Three to Six, they have arisen without their wider implications being recognised and without a vision as to how they should fit together in a coherent whole. As a result, a series of new tasks remain to be addressed systematically, some of which fall to the Centre and some to the local NHS.

Our analysis suggests that the central role comprises:

- defining and designing systems of care
- devising system rules and aligning incentives, and determining how service structure and service organisation should be linked defining the rules, particularly those governing professional activity

- regulation, monitoring, accountability and audit for systems of care
- linking service delivery and design with other health care functions, particularly training and workforce planning
- ensuring the knowledge base
- managing systems of care and ensuring overall consistency and coherence between the policies adopted in all parts of the health care delivery system.

Having looked briefly at each of these, we then consider some issues that arise at local level.

The design of systems of care

It may seem self-evident that in an organisation such as the NHS the Centre should take the leading role in service design. Even in a less-centralised health care delivery system, there would be an obvious case for entrusting that task to one agency, simply on the grounds of economising on the effort of gathering all the relevant information about costs, user needs and clinical effectiveness.

The argument for proceeding in this way is all the stronger for small care systems, such as for cleft lip/palette,[1] which even referring clinicians may know little about, and for care systems where the clientele differs little from area to area and not in such a way as to undermine a common approach to service delivery.

But while these arguments are strong, and have been more or less taken for granted within the UK in the process of developing national service frameworks, they are not always compelling. As pointed out in Chapter Eight, the knowledge base underpinning systems of care is weak. Cancer apart, the UK has no national disease database, while in all areas many of the key elements of system design are missing. Consequently, there is, generally speaking, no 'best' system of delivery. And even if there were, new data and clinical innovation would redefine what was originally found to be best.

Furthermore, a great deal of the evidence on the effectiveness of different ways of delivering care comes from specific instances of successful delivery. In the case of the mental illness national service framework, a number of examples of 'good practice' are cited that reflect experience in particular areas. These may not be transferable, or at least not without modification in the light of different local circumstances.

The central role, therefore, may best be described as supportive in a number of key areas, principally the assimilation of relevant data and research, the design of key components such as minimum data sets, the exchange of comparative information on performance, and the design of, or support for, experiments in new ways of delivering services.[2]

The national service frameworks for coronary heart disease and for mental health each identify the need for extensive programmes of technical work, as noted in the previous chapter, and these areas have been recognised as priorities for NHS R&D monies. These proposals imply, correctly, that the design process should be seen as a continuing activity.

Over and above tasks focused on specific systems of care, there is a further role for the Centre – the design of the whole delivery system. The 'model' of health care delivery we have built up is one of a series of interconnecting and at times conflicting pathways or systems of care. We noted in Chapters Four, Five and Seven that there are different ways of breaking down the whole care system into systems of care: at the moment the choice between them is never explicitly made. Any attempt to do so would founder on lack of research on alternative structures and inadequate descriptive information of what happens now.

The central role should, therefore, not be to define a whole care delivery system in precise terms, but rather to promote debate and reflection about the possible options and to encourage experiment and research in areas that are critical to the evaluation of those options. The programme of national service frameworks will eventually force these structural issues to the surface, but as far as we are aware they are being developed in isolation, without any attempt to identify the issues their overall development will raise. But if 'the whole system' is to mean what it says, some attempt to fit the various systems of care together must be made.

Defining the rules

In any national health service funded from a common source, some nationally imposed rules are inevitable, if only to meet the basic requirements of accountability. But once these basic requirements are satisfied, it is less clear how far standardisation should go. Equity between areas argues one way, the need for experiment and innovation the other. However that issue is decided, the scope for local discretion will be centrally determined. The areas we consider next, therefore, fall to the Centre to decide on, though that decision may entail the creation of local discretion.

The financial framework

The vast bulk of the financial resources of the NHS are allocated as a block or general grant. The Government, however, is making extensive use of targeted funds[3] for services, such as cancer and heart disease, for which national service frameworks exist. As it stands, this approach cannot ensure any particular level of funding for each system since the targeted funds represent only a fraction of total spending. It is arguable, however, in the light of the conclusions of Chapter Seven, that each framework should be separately funded.

The notion that resource allocation should be linked to systems of care stems naturally from developments in public sector budgeting in the 1960s. The idea was floated and partially implemented in the 1970s, following the issue of *Priorities for Health and Personal Social Services in England.*[4] In the event, the Centre did not have the will or the confidence to impose its view of priorities. It has been developed at local level in a few parts of the NHS.[5]

If variations in local epidemiology were such as to render infeasible a nationally set local budget for each care system, a case would remain for using the system of care as a financial reporting framework – and *that* could reasonably be a central requirement. In fact, the guidance issued for the development of health improvement programmes[6] requires that they should comprise a service and financial framework setting out 'in broad terms how resources are to be allocated to meet national and related priorities'. This could be the start of moving towards a system of care budgeting process at local level and reporting at national level.

The central argument for going down this path is one of accountability. The system of care provides an obvious way of showing, to both the public and the Centre, what purchasers are doing with the resources available to them.

We noted in the first part of this book that the separation of funding into two main streams – the main financial obstacle to the development of systems of care within the NHS – has been removed. But, helpful though this may be, it is insufficient in itself. A basic requirement is that costs should be available for care pathways within and between organisations. While it is up to the local NHS to derive them, there is a role for the Centre in trying to ensure that the capacity to do so exists. That capacity does not yet exist across the board.

A further technical requirement is that financial structures should allow for interdependencies between care systems over time. As we showed in Chapter

Four, these interdependencies are of various kinds, each of which poses its own requirements on the financial system. Unless these interdependencies are understood, however, the financial framework cannot be correctly set.

Financial frameworks are largely if not wholly geared to annual financial reporting. But as pointed out in Chapter Eight, many of the key relationships between and within care systems are long term. On the provider side, much of health capital is long lived and hence resources cannot be shifted quickly: only a long planning horizon will reveal whether a shift from hospital to community is justified on cost grounds. On the demand side, the interactions between social care and health care are potentially of critical importance, as the example taken from the work of the Audit Commission showed (Table 8.1), but their scale and nature is not understood. For example, the links between preventive or anticipatory policies designed to forestall future health and social care problems require long term monitoring if they are to be established and their scale measured. That would require longitudinal monitoring of large numbers of people of a kind carried out, for example, for the national cohort studies,[7] but of a more frequent and targeted nature.

Such work, even if started now, would take years to produce useful results. But there may be scope for using the annual NHS user surveys,[8] if designed with these requirements in mind, to identify whether, for example, patterns of social care delivery and emergency hospitals admissions were correlated. As far as we are aware, however, systematic attempts to link this kind of work with financial systems have yet to begin.

The organisational framework

In Chapter Seven, we pointed to the tensions arising from the development of systems of care and an organisational structure based on provider organisations that operate within a similar set of rules.

Within a national health service, it is a reasonable expectation that its constituent bodies should be subject to similar rules, at least as long as they remain fully within the public sector, particularly those relating to financial and clinical accountability, and relations with users and the public at large. There are other technical areas, such as data collection, that should be common.

Our analysis has also suggested that it is hard to determine where the formal boundaries of organisations should be set, given the scope for 'organisation' stemming from the use of clinical rules and contractual links between providers. What the right balance between these integrating devices should be remains to be worked out for all the elements of the health care delivery system.

For the same reason, there is a case, as suggested in Chapter Seven, for permitting the creation of trusts on different bases, including clinically defined and managed trusts covering systems of care and some contributing services, as envisaged, for example, in the option proposed for emergency services by the New Health Network.[9] Our analysis suggests there may be benefits in this approach, but it also suggests that any such change would raise a new set of issues around access to the resources shared with other systems of care. The way forward, therefore, is through local experiment.[10]

Defining professional roles

At no time during the life of the NHS have all the factors bearing on the structure of the workforce as a whole been considered together. As the HSMU report[11] put it:

- *there is no mechanism for drawing together separate streams of development or reviewing them from a wider service perspective …;*
- *the healthcare workforce is organised in a wide range of occupations and separate specialisms within these occupations. The complexity of the structure complicates the planning process and can be a constraint on the re-alignment of services;*
- *the fragmentation of the workforce makes the development of supply plans more difficult so that, even in periods of high unemployment, the NHS has difficulty in recruiting to some occupations;*
- *one of the biggest problems is the inflexibility which is the inevitable consequence of having to plan and manage such a wide range of occupations.* (p 75)

We noted above the Health Committee's report on NHS staffing requirements, which recommended:

> … *a major review of current planning procedures which should pay particular regard to their rationalisation and eventual replacement by an integrated planning system. We think it necessary that any new system should not only incorporate the national overview currently provided by the sub-group of the NHSE, but also actively promote a national strategy for workforce planning which, allowing for local conditions, brings a sense of consistency and cohesion at present notable for its absence.* (para 36, p 5)

The Government response led in due course to the establishment of a review. The resulting report[12] made a number of proposals bearing on the issues discussed in this chapter, and identified a large number of weaknesses in existing arrangements. The length of the list (see Box 9.1) indicates just how much there is to be done.

Although this review moves the argument in the right direction, despite the range and radical nature of its proposals[13] it still falls short of what is required. In

Box 9.1 Weaknesses in workforce planning

- *greater attention needs to be paid to making proper links between service, finance and workforce planning both at local and national level;*
- *the approaches to workforce planning for doctors and dentists and for other clinical staff are not aligned;*
- *there is also insufficient recognition of the role of non-NHS employers in work-force planning and development;*
- *... separation of funding streams. The main levies (SIFT, MADEL, and NMET) and other sources of funding from NHS Trusts or other bodies to support workforce development in its broadest sense, including library and IT provision, are managed as separate pockets of money;*
- *there are major weaknesses in the information base used for workforce planning;*
- *the lack of a consistent effort to build research and development findings into thinking about the future workforce;*
- *the lack of a consistent focus on skill-mix issues;*
- *no national drive to share learning and good practice or to support NHS Trusts seeking to develop innovative approaches;*
- *this needs to change if the NHS is to deliver the sort of service which Ministers want to see;*
- *a shortage of technical planning skills;*
- *the perceived pressure on young professionals to settle on their careers at an early stage in their training;*
- *the potential impact of specialisation on the ability to run effective services e.g. to establish appropriate surgical 'on-take' arrangements;*
- *there is also insufficient support for staff who wish to change roles during a health-care career.* (pp 20–1)

... we believe that workforce planning and development is not embedded in the culture of the NHS, with too much short-term crisis handling and a lack of constant attention to the impact of many day-to-day decisions on the workforce of the future. (p 25)

Source: Department of Health, 2000d.

particular, it fails to address the core issue, discussed in Chapter Five, of how to relate workforce and service planning at the most fundamental levels, such as the definitions of the professions themselves and the impact of the development of care systems on the characteristics of the workforce required by the health care delivery system.

It thus fails to mesh with the other elements required to define the scope and nature of professional roles. Although it argued for the removal of barriers across professional boundaries, it did not address the basis of specialisation and the links between that and the efficient delivery of services. It also failed to acknowledge the changes actually, as well as potentially, taking place in the pattern of service delivery. As we noted, the creation of systems of care requires a change in focus on the part of the individual professional, while their design and management require new skills that are not normally found among clinicians (at least not as part of their formal training). We turn to this issue in the next section.

Managing systems of care

The 'vision' of the care delivery system built up in the previous chapter is one of a series of interlocking pathways and systems of care. The main consequence of focusing on systems of care is that service delivery must be designed, planned and delivered across existing boundaries of responsibility, with or between organisations. Furthermore, because the characteristics of each system are likely to be different, they will not simply nest inside or alongside each other within one regional health care delivery system. The hospital emerges, above all, as the place where a number of systems coincide because of their common need for its facilities and support services. The community displays similar conflicts, with different professional groups contributing to more than one care system. There will be continuing boundary 'conflicts' that require resolution.

The NHS has run on a system of 'management without management', designed to maintain clinical discretion. It is one of the most curious elements of health care systems that they operate largely without anyone in charge and do so more or less effectively on a day-to-day basis.

That they do so is a reflection of the force of convention. Patients flow from one part of the system along accustomed pathways in more or less predictable ways. The development of care protocols, etc., have been designed to make such informal processes more regular and predictable. But the question of enforcement or, as it would now be called, 'governance', has for most of the life of the NHS been ignored. Against this background, it not surprising that guidelines and protocols have been more honoured in the breach than in the observance.[14]

The development of care pathways and programmes of care is an attempt to impose order on these processes; doing so requires a co-operative effort. But once the care pathway or the care system is in place, the question remains of who is in charge. This question is rarely addressed directly.

As we saw in the citations from the Scottish circular (see page 131) the term 'clinical leadership' is used in recognition of the need for management. But while leadership is clearly important as a means to set up a network, it does not provide the basis for accountability for day-to-day performance. The national service frameworks do not tackle this issue directly. The Government has appointed so-called cancer and heart disease 'tsars' for the English national service frameworks, but these have no formal powers over the clinicians and others involved.

Given the geographical scale of the major systems of care and the range of organisations from which they draw, it would make sense for them to be managed centrally, or through 'subsidiaries' of the Centre, such as regions. Clearly the larger the care system in geographical and population terms, the stronger the case for this approach. It would be all the stronger if care systems were to achieve, as suggested in Chapter Seven, some degree of organisational independence.

Whether this approach is adopted or not, the interfaces between systems where they use the same physical or human assets also require management. This could be a regional/local role or a central one, depending on where the key interdependencies were to be found. For example, if they arose within the medical workforce, central action may be appropriate, but if within the physical structure, local action might be.

However this is decided, there remains an overall task of system management – falling in the UK to the Centre. This has two aspects: first, monitoring the performance of systems of care; and second, the interaction of care with the other functions of the NHS, principally training and research.

Given the size of the NHS, there must be some devolution within it. The NHS Plan acknowledges this and proposes a new arrangement for earned devolution based on a classification of NHS organisations into red (failing), yellow (failing in some respects) and green (outstanding performance) (para 6.26).

Against the background of the current analysis, this emphasis on institutions is inappropriate, and reflects an incomplete understanding of the other changes the Government has been promoting. If systems of care are adopted as the key structural element of the whole system, then it is these that should be the object of performance monitoring. The focus on the existing formal organisations is misplaced.

The same is true of performance measures. The present UK Government has placed greater emphasis than any of its predecessors on the use of performance indicators to judge NHS performance, specifically through its national performance assessment framework, and, within the national service framework documents, each care system.

The first of these does not fit well with the analytic approach adopted here. This suggests that to test system performance requires a number of indicators that do not emerge from considering specific treatment activities:

- because they are concerned with routing decisions at interfaces
- because success requires contributions from more than one provider
- because judgements are required on the extent to which overall performance is affected by factors outside the health care delivery system.

The first point has been recognised to some extent. The NHS performance indicators set contains some bearing on interfaces and the first NHS national user survey has asked relevant questions on the interface between GP and hospital.

But the other issues underlying the assessment of performance have scarcely been tackled at all. In particular, the conceptual frameworks required for assessing systems of care delivery in the context of the whole system of care of which they form part, and the context in which they operate, are only just being developed. As we argued in the previous chapter, unless these are clarified, the balance between different interventions and between care interventions and other measures cannot be determined. Getting this balance right is perhaps *the* central strategic issue for a Department of Health running a national health service.[15]

The second task is to ensure that the overall interest is served, through a principled reconciliation of the different interests – training, research and care delivery – that meet within the health care delivery system. The Department of Health does not have responsibility for all the elements. But unless these various interests are reconciled, particularly training with service delivery, whatever independent view of the future of the whole delivery system is arrived at may not be realisable because the 'bundles' of skills being produced by the medical education system do not match those required by the care delivery system, and hence some options desirable for the delivery of care cannot be implemented.

Essentially the same arguments apply to research. For some years now, the Department of Health has supported a Health Technology Assessment Programme that contains an element of 'horizon scanning'. While this is valuable, it addresses only one element among many that will shape the way health care is delivered in the future.[16] No-one can predict these with confidence: the central role here is to provide directly, or ensure through suitably supported research, a continuous monitoring of trends and new developments likely to change the way health care is delivered, and an assessment of their potential significance for the overall structure as well as its components – the systems of care. It is particularly important that such monitoring should focus on factors that might undermine the existing set of systems of care by suggesting that some should be merged or that new ones should be created.

Accountability and audit

We concluded in Chapter Seven that it was not generally possible to align formal organisational structures with systems of care and recent official publications supporting, for example, managed clinical networks make a positive virtue of this feature. But it is these formal structures that provide the basis for the accountability of the Service, including its audit.

The external audit arrangements for the NHS – the Audit Commission and the National Audit Office – are not well suited to the broad remit that systems of care require. The audit bodies have made it clear that they are aware that current arrangements are not adequate.[17] Furthermore, the Audit Commission and the Commission for Health Improvement have joined forces to monitor the implementation of the NHS Cancer Plan.

In particular areas, both value-for-money auditing and inspection have attempted to bridge boundaries between public sector bodies; the Audit Commission reports on children's services and care for elderly people have straddled health and social care.

But such a process cannot address those areas where private and voluntary bodies are involved – both important for many with continuing care needs – and it cannot tackle the issues arising from the interplay of the system of care with the broader environment. The audit of a system of care delivery, in other words, must adopt a wider view of the relevant system and take all the major outside influences into account.[18] That step has yet to be taken.

Implementation: the local dimension

However large the role of the Centre, the task of actually creating systems of care must fall to localities – with the exception of the relatively few services that are commissioned nationally. The absorption of the information and guidelines contained in the national service framework documents is a massive task in itself, but it is essentially a familiar one. The creation of a system of care, however, as we argued in Chapter Three, poses new requirements of which the most basic are the ability to 'see the whole' and to understand how the parts fit together and how it works in practice.

As we argued above, the information base is currently poor, but if a start is to be made at local level, then the best has to be made of what does exist. We consider some relevant techniques first. We then go on to discuss techniques that attempt to overcome some of the structural obstacles.

Understanding the local system

The starting point for the design of a system of care is the population it is intended to serve. But, as has already been pointed out, information on the incidence of even common conditions such as stroke is poor.

Recognising this in relation to care for elderly people, the Audit Commission proposed that authorities should map the services in their area. As this report indicates, the technique is a useful, if traditional, way of conducting a stock stake of the current situation. The next step is to map the flows of users between services. Despite the developments within the NHS designed to improve emergency planning, such information is very rare. Furthermore, even the existing data, e.g. on the use of hospitals, are rarely analysed in a systematic and useful way. And as noted in the previous chapter, local registers of people with particular conditions are also rare.[19] Although these will develop in time, in general the basis for simple descriptions of patient flows through a whole care system does not yet exist. While the Centre may support and advise, the mapping itself must be a local task.

Creating a local system

The creation of systems of care requires a mutual recognition of membership and a willingness to work within a common framework. The vast UK experience of trying to make effective links between hospital and community, and between health and social care more generally, indicates that these conditions often do not hold.

Even the relatively limited task of defining a care pathway, in practice, requires sustained co-operative working by professionals with different backgrounds, many of whom already know each other.[20] Experience show this can be difficult, even where the pathway involves only a small 'slice' out of the activity of a hospital since, even in that limited context, a range of different interests has to be reconciled.[21]

The task becomes several times more difficult when different organisations are involved and where there may be no recognition, at least on a day-to-day basis, that they each contribute to a particular system of care. As we have argued in Chapter Seven, cross-boundary working is inevitable and so means must be devised to support it. The various measures taken by the present Government[22] recognise this. But to make them work requires substantial investment in mutual learning across all the boundaries that tend to balkanise health care delivery: organisation, profession, finance.

Processes have been devised which promote the sense of mutual belonging that a system of care implies. As Pratt and colleagues[23] put it:

> *The behaviour of the system depends on the way the parts are connected as well as the way the parts themselves behave. Success is dependent on the mutually appropriate development of the constituent parts.* (p 12)

As their work makes clear, this 'whole systems' approach is not meant to be one-off. It may be possible to resolve difficulties over particular interfaces, such as hospital discharge by a once-and-for-all agreement, but whole systems of care cannot be treated in this way. There has to be a continuing forum for interchange and a continuing collaborative framework running across different organisations.

Such a framework must have some kind of administrative element. But it can be supported by the simulation and other modelling techniques referred to in the previous chapter. The advantage of a model, even when not used for forecasting, is that it forces assumptions and gaps out into the open, and thereby assists the components of the whole system to reach a shared understanding of how the system works. In this way, it provides a basis for joint learning on the part of representatives of different components of a system of care.[24]

Facility planning

The simple, and obvious, implication of our framework of analysis is that the planning of a specific physical facility designed to provide one element of a system of care should be set against the wider system of which it forms part. If care systems were separate from each other, that would be relatively straightforward. But inevitably, because of the interconnections discussed in Chapter Three, some decisions have to be made for a series of systems at one and the same time. This is particularly true of hospitals, given the wide range of support and clinical services they embody.

As we have suggested above, hospitals should be seen as the place where a number of not otherwise all-that-closely related pathways come together, because of the need to use joint facilities or because of other presumed benefits of spatial contiguity. So, while the hospital as a physical asset requires planning in its own right, it follows from our analysis that the planning process for hospitals is part of the planning process of each care system.

In the past, the typical hospital forecasting model ignored this, concentrating simply on projections of bed use on the basis of past trends in overall use and length of stay. The report of the National Beds Inquiry[25] did adopt a 'whole systems' approach, if only in part. Its central argument is that the bulk of hospital bed days are 'consumed' by elderly people and hence that planning for hospitals should comprise planning elderly care. Although this represents a step in the right direction, it is incomplete. The logic of the report of the National Beds Inquiry's treatment of care for the elderly applies equally strongly to emergency care and paediatrics, and less so to other care systems. Accordingly, local infrastructure should be planned at the whole (local) system level so as to allow all elements of the pathways running across hospital and community boundaries to be taken into account. While there are signs this is being recognised,[26] in general the need for this has yet to be acknowledged at either central or local level.[27]

Conclusion

The NHS is slowly moving in the direction of developing systems of care, but its implications for the overall management of the system and for service development at local level have yet to be appreciated. In particular:

- there are outstanding and major technical issues to be resolved, above all the development of appropriate statistical systems that lag behind the development of care systems
- the management of the system remains focused on existing organisations, as do the wider arrangements for accountability and audit
- there is no framework for bringing together all the relevant elements and ensuring (or trying to ensure) their consistency.

In other words, while those currently responsible for the NHS as a whole are beginning to make many of the relevant connections between the different policy areas that impinge on service delivery, they have yet to grasp the full implications of the developments they are currently promoting for service delivery and face up to the interdependence and complexity that typifies the NHS, like any other health care delivery system.

That said, there is no ready solution to the problems and difficulties we have identified. Indeed, the notion of a solution or 'best system' is misguided. The forces making for change in health care delivery systems worldwide – technological advance, financial constraints, consumer expectations and the social and political framework into which health care systems fit – are not predictable, except in the sense that it is certain they will continue to create a need for further change. What those 'in charge' can do, however, is consider how the existing system of care delivery is best structured to deal with change by reducing the strength of the existing barriers to it and by avoiding, where possible, major investments in resources, human or otherwise, that cannot readily be moved to other uses.

References

1. See the Clinical Standards Advisory Group report (1998b), which revealed how poorly this service was designed. Since its publication, steps have been taken to remedy this.
2. Examples of all these can be found in the programmes of work defined by the national service frameworks and the NHS Cancer Plan.
3. See Appleby, 1999.

4. Department of Health and Social Security, 1976.
5. See, for example, Craig *et al.*, 1995. Monaghan *et al.*, 1999, suggest that individual managed clinical networks should have their own budgets. Oni, 1996, proposes that consultants should be budget holders.
6. Department of Health, 1998c.
7. Pringle, 1966.
8. Airey and Erens, 1999.
9. Coffey and Mythen, 2000.
10. In a sense, the NHS has been here before, with the experiments with clinical budgeting carried out in the 1980s. However, these budgets were set within hospitals only but the experience (see Packwood *et al.*, 1991) is relevant nonetheless.
11. Health Service Management Unit,1996.
12. Department of Health, 2000d.
13. Doyal and Cameron, 2000, point out that:

    By its very nature the healthcare labour force is an interdependent one. The different occupational groups did not develop in isolation from each other but as part of a complex and interdependent system capable of carrying out the many activities that make up a modern health service. Yet despite this obvious reciprocity, the different elements of the NHS labour force are still planned and managed in isolation. This continuing fragmentation has a major impact on the quality of patient care and on the wellbeing of health workers themselves.
14. See, for example, Day, 1999; House of Commons, 1999.
15. One that it has failed to tackle in relation to breast cancer screening; see Mulligan, 2000a.
16. See, for example, the consultation paper on the research needs of the NHS (Department of Health, 2000e) and the King's Fund comments on it (available from the author or the Fund's web site).
17. Public Audit Form, 1999.
18. Mulligan, 2000b.
19. Some GP practices have them, but the picture is patchy.
20. See Weiner, 2000.
21. See, for example, Johnson, 1997.
22. See Chapter Two.
23. Pratt *et al.*, 1999.
24. Cropper and Forte, 1997.
25. Department of Health, 2000g.
26. See, for example, NHS Wales, 2000.
27. As we have argued elsewhere (Boyle and Harrison, 2000a & b), the commissioning of hospitals should not be left to hospital trusts alone precisely because of their limited remit. This point is well made in NHS Wales, 2000.

Chapter Ten

Overview

The question posed in the thought experiment with which we began has not been answered. Rather, it has led to the identification of a series of interlocking considerations bearing on professional roles, the role of users, the tensions between alternative definitions of the scope of systems of care, and the proper role for formal organisation. Of necessity we have had to consider these one at a time. The challenge for those thinking about the future of health care delivery is to maintain a debate that keeps all of them in play at one and the same time and to make the connections between them effective in practice.

Our brief historical survey of the main threads of the various attempts made over decades to improve the structure of the NHS, in the broad sense defined here, concluded that so far that challenge had not been met. The reason is not hard to determine – the complexity of health care delivery.

This complexity stems not simply from the range of issues it encompasses, but also the nature and extent of the interconnections between the various elements it comprises, between the health care system as a whole and individual care systems, and between these and the wider physical social and economic environment.

The notion of a system provides a way of identifying the nature of these interconnections and the nature of the gaps in current knowledge that hinder the development of particular systems of care. But the notion of a system is simultaneously helpful and disabling, emphasising, as it does, how hard it is to find a solid base of knowledge on which to build a structure even at the level of theory. The very arguments that lead to regarding the health care delivery system as a series of systems of care undermine attempts to understand, forecast and plan for it.

Everything, or nearly everything connects, usually in ways that are poorly recorded and, where recorded, poorly understood. There can be no general presumption that improving one pathway will improve the health care delivery system as a whole.

This may seem both a counsel of despair and totally impractical. The capacity to understand the whole does not exist and never will do. Hands-on knowledge of how things work now soon becomes out of date as society and technology changes. In practice, reform or service development change must always be incremental and partial. Yet, as we have argued, that approach is inherently risky.

This book has acknowledged that that change must in practice be incremental and partial, but it has argued that considering the wider context in which any part of the health care delivery sits has two merits:

- It identifies issues and areas which can be illuminated by research and other forms of intelligence that the incremental approach fails to identify.
- It may contribute to pinning down those circumstances where incrementalism is enough, and those where it is not.

As we noted at several points in this book, the bulk of the effort devoted to improving health care delivery lies at the level of the specific intervention, the micro end of the spectrum where the provider based care pathway also belongs. The other end of the spectrum, the macro end, is not so well researched. Despite the vast amount of change that has been visited on the NHS, the underlying structure of service delivery has usually been ignored. White Papers have come and gone in the past 20 years with scarcely a mention of the factors changing the health care delivery system independently of the changes they have proposed. The hospital has been virtually invisible in official papers. Professional documents have kept firmly to their professional boundaries. Seeing 'the whole' continues to be more honoured in the breach than in the observance.

The Service needs a strategic capacity. This capacity should not and could not attempt to foresee every possible change, nor should it draw up a masterplan for service delivery. Rather, it should focus on the connections between the main issues we have considered here – professional roles, service structures and organisational roles – as well as some we have not, particularly the linkages between clinical research, medical training and the role of hospitals. To gain perspective the UK NHS needs to have available to it a much greater capacity for international cross-system comparisons of delivery mechanisms.

Systems of care fall firmly into the middle ground between trying to see the 'whole of the whole' and focusing on the specific clinical encounter. Until recently, this middle ground was also neglected: now it is slowly being explored. The developments described in Chapter Two represent a growing realisation that the way health care is delivered on the ground requires sustained analytic, clinical and managerial attention at a level broader than the 'micro' focus that has typified the Service in the past.

While these developments are welcome, they represent a starting point rather than a conclusion. Our analysis suggests that a large number of difficult technical tasks remain, of which the most central are:

- greater understanding of the interaction between users and care systems. In *The NHS: Facing the Future*, we suggested that every policy proposal should be accompanied by a demand audit, a recommendation that the NHS Plan conspicuously disregarded
- sustained development of professional roles, particularly in cross-cutting systems of care such as emergencies, is required as part of a broader effort to understand how systems of care, defined conventionally or by new criteria, interact with each other
- consideration needs to be given to which steps should be taken to ensure that knowledge matches the direction in which policy is slowly pushing the NHS, and the gaps that make themselves evident once sustained attention is given to service delivery and the management of performance at the system level are filled.
- the organisational framework, including performance monitoring, auditing and accountability, needs to be adjusted to take into account those systems of care that do not fit organisational boundaries.

This is a large agenda but, as noted in various parts of this book, a start been made on it. The need now is to pursue it more energetically.

Bibliography

Airey C, Erens B, editors. *National surveys of NHS patients. General practice 1998.* London: NHS Executive, 1999.

Anderson L. The introduction of generic workers into the ward team: an explanatory study. *Journal of Nursing Management* 1997; 5: 69–75.

Appleby J. The modernisation fund. In: *Health Care UK 1999/2000*. London: King's Fund, 1999.

Armstrong P. The role of the clinical nurse specialist. *Nursing Standard* 1999; 13 (16): 40–2.

Audit Commission. *Seen but not heard: co-ordinating community child health and social services for children in need*. London: Audit Commission, 1994.

Audit Commission. *United they stand: co-ordinating care for elderly patients with hip fracture*. London: HMSO, 1995.

Audit Commission. *What the doctor ordered: a study of GP fundholders in England and Wales*. London: HMSO, 1996a.

Audit Commission. *By accident or design: improving A&E services in England and Wales.* London: Audit Commission, 1996b.

Audit Commission. *The coming of age*. London: Audit Commission, 1997a.

Audit Commission. *Anaesthesia under examination: the efficiency and effectiveness of anaesthesia and pain relief services in England and Wales*. London: Audit Commission, 1997b.

Audit Commission. *Reports and accounts: year ending 31 March 1999*. London: Audit Commission, 1999a.

Audit Commission. *Children in mind: child and adolescent mental health services*. London: Audit Commission, 1999b.

Audit Commission. *Critical to success: the place of efficient and effective critical care services within the acute hospital*. London: Audit Commission, 1999c.

Audit Commission. *Testing times: a review of diabetes services in England and Wales.* London: Audit Commission, 2000a.

Audit Commission. *The way to go home: rehabilitation and remedial services for older people.* London: Audit Commission, 2000b.

Baker R, Preston C, Cheater F, Hearnshaw H. Measuring patients' attitudes to care across the primary/secondary interface: the development of the patient carer diary. *Quality in Health Care* 1999; 8: 154–60.

Baker R. Will the future GP remain a personal doctor? *British Journal of General Practice* 1997; 47: 831–4.

Banks T. The French way: emergency health care provision. *Accident and Emergency Nursing* 1998; 6: 197–9.

Barnes J, Smith R. Why healthcare systems need medical managers. *BMJ* 1997; 314: 1636–7.

Bechel D L, Myers W A, Smith D G. Does patient-centred care pay off? *Journal on Quality Improvement* 2000; 26 (7): 400–9.

Beddard F D *et al. Positions, movements and directions in health services research.* Oxford: Oxford University Press, 1974.

Berino E *et al.*, editors. *Eurocare 2: survival of cancer patients in Europe in the late eighties.* Lyon, France: IARC, 1999.

Berwick D. Medical associations: guilds or leaders. *BMJ* 1997; 314: 1564–5.

Billings J, Wells F C. Delays in the diagnosis and surgical treatment of lung cancer. *Thorax* 1996; September: 903–6.

Black D, Bowman C. Community institutional care for frail elderly people. *BMJ* 1997; 315: 441–2.

Boaden N. *Primary care: making connections.* Buckingham: Open University Press, 1997.

Bodenheimer T. Disease management in the American market. *BMJ* 2000; 320: 563–6.

Bodenheimer T, Lo B, Casalino L. Primary care physicians should be coordinators, not gatekeepers. *JAMA* 1999; 281 (21): 2045–9.

Boerma W G W, van der Zee J, Fleming D M. Service profiles of general practitioners in Europe. *British Journal of General Practice*, 1997; 47: 481–6.

Bosanquet N, Franks P. *Stroke care: reducing the burden of disease.* London: The Stroke Association, 1998.

Boyle S, Bryan-Jones J, Harrison A, Tansley J. *Packaging systems thoughts for managers to use.* Paper presented to European Healthcare Management Association Conference, Trinity College, Dublin, 24–26 June 1998. Session 9: Healthcare management education and organisation development.

Boyle S, Harrison A. Private finance and service development. In: *Health Care UK Autumn 2000.* London: King's Fund, 2000a.

Boyle S, Harrison A. PFI in health: the story so far. In: Kelly G, Robinson P, editors. *A healthy partnership: the future of public private partnerships in the health service.* London: IPPR, 2000b.

Boyle S, Bryan-Jones J, Harrison A, Tansley J. *The urgent care system.* Unpublished paper, available from author.

Bradley C, Blenkinsopp A. The future for self medication. *BMJ* 1996: 312: 835–7.

Brampton S. A patient's perspective of continuity. *BMJ* 2000; 321: 735–6.

British Market Research Bureau. *Everyday health care: a consumer study of self-medication in Great Britain*. London: BMRB, 1997.

British Medical Association, Central Consultants and Specialists Committee. *Towards tomorrow: the future role of the consultant*. London: BMA, 1996.

British Medical Association, Health Policy and Economic Research Unit. *Leaner and fitter*. London: BMA, 1997.

British Medical Association, Royal College of Physicians of London, Royal College of Surgeons of England. *Provision of acute general hospital services*. London: BMA, 1998.

Broadbent J, Dietrich M, Roberts J. *The end of the professions?* London: Routledge, 1997.

Bruster S, Jarman B, Bosanquet N, Weston D, Erens R, Delbanco T L. National survey of hospital patients. *BMJ* 1994; 309: 1542–6.

Buck D, Eastwood A, Smith P C. Can we measure the social importance of health care? *International Journal of Technology Assessment in Health Care* 1999; 15 (1): 89–107.

Bull M J. Discharge planning for older people: a review of current research. *British Journal of Community Nursing* 2000; 5: 70–4.

Cancer Research Campaign, King's Fund, Macmillan Cancer Relief. *The workforce and training implications of the Calman/Hine cancer report*. London: The Cancer Collaboration, 1997.

Chartered Society of Physiotherapy. *Chartered physiotherapists working as extended scope practitioners*. London: The Chartered Society of Physiotherapy, 2000.

Clark N M, Gong M. Management of chronic disease by practitioners and patients: are we teaching the wrong things? *BMJ* 2000; 320: 572–5.

Clinical Standards Advisory Group. *Standards of clinical care for people with diabetes*. London: HMSO, 1994.

Clinical Standards Advisory Group. *Community health care for elderly people: report of a CSAG committee*. London: TSO, 1998a.

Clinical Standards Advisory Group. *Cleft lip and/or palate: report of a CSAG committee*. London: TSO, 1998b.

Clinical Standards Advisory Group. *Services for patients with pain*. London: Department of Health, 2000.

Coats T J, Goode A. Opportunity to improve pre-hospital care in the UK. *Lancet* 1999; 353: 1292.

Coeberg J W W, Janssen-Heijnen M L G, Post P N, Razenberg P P A. Serious co-morbidity among unselected cancer patients newly diagnosed in the southeastern part of The Netherlands in 1993–1996. *Journal of Clinical Epidemiology* 1999; 52 (12): 1131–6.

Coffey T, Mythen M, editors. *NHS Frontline – visions for 2010*. London: The New Health Network, 2000.

Coleman E A, Grothaus L C, Sandhu N, Wagner E H. Chronic care clinics: a randomized controlled trial of a new model of primary care for frail older adults. *Journal of the American Geriatrics Society* 1999; 47: 775–83.

Connor H. Who needs a general physician? *Journal of the Royal College of Physicians of London* 1998; 32 (6): 548–51.

Cook R I, Render M, Woods D. Gaps in the continuity of care and progress on patient safety. *BMJ* 2000; 320: 791–4.

Court S D M, chair. *Fit for the future: report of the committee on child health services. Vol. 1*. London: HMSO, 1976.

Craft I *et al*. *Specialized futures: essays in honour of Sir George Godber GCB*. London: Oxford University Press for the Nuffield Provincial Hospitals Trust, 1975.

Craig G. The case for widening the referral system. *Journal of the Royal College of Physicians of London* 1996; 30: 80–2.

Craig J. *Changing childbirth*. London: HMSO, 1993.

Craig N, Parkin D, Gerard K. Clearing the fog on the Tyne: programme budgeting in Newcastle and North Tyneside Health Authority. *Health Policy* 1995; 33: 107–25.

Craig R, Dale J. Telephone triage. Part 1: identifying the demand. *Nursing Standard* 1998; 12 (34): 33–8.

Cropper S, Forte P, editors. *Enhancing health services management. The role of decision support systems*. Buckingham: Open University Press, 1997.

Crouch R, Dale J. Telephone triage. Part 2: how good are the decisions? *Nursing Standard* 1998; 12 (35): 33–9.

Culyer A, chair. *Supporting research and development in the NHS. Report of the task force*. London: HMSO, 1994.

Cumberlege J. *Changing childbirth: the Cumberlege Report*. London: HMSO, 1993.

Currie C. *Audit based simulation of hip fracture care to explore major policy options, responses to demographic change and impact of generalisation of best practice guidelines*. National Research Register project N0470026917, 2000.

David A S. *Determinants of delay seeking treatment for breast symptoms*. London: Institute of Psychiatry, 1997.

Davies C. *General practitioner open access to diagnostic services for cancer*. Coventry: Warwick Business School, 1999.

Davis R M, Wagner E G, Groves T. Advances in managing chronic disease. *BMJ* 2000; 320: 525–6.

Dawson, Lord, chair. *The Dawson report on the future provision of medical and allied services: an interim report by the consultative council on medical and allied services*. London: HMSO, 1920; reprinted London: King Edward's Hospital Fund for London, 1950.

Day P, Klein R, Miller F. *Hurdles and levers: a comparative US–UK study of guidelines*. London: Nuffield Trust, 1998.

de Bono D. Development and future of open access echocardiography. *Hospital Medicine* 1998; 59 (8): 600–2.

de Luc K. Are different models of care pathways being developed? *International Journal of Health Care Quality Assurance* 2000; 13 (2): 80–6.

Dennis T, Owens D. Transforming local care. *Journal of Telemedicine and Telecare* 2000; 6: 102–3.

Department of Health. *Self-governing hospitals: an initial guide*. London: HMSO, 1989.

Department of Health. *Research for health*. London: HMSO, 1991.

Department of Health. *Planning the medical workforce. Medical Manpower Standing Advisory Committee: first report*. London: HMSO, 1992.

Department of Health. *Planning the medical workforce. Medical Workforce Standing Advisory Committee: second report*. London: HMSO, 1995.

Department of Health. *In the patient's interest: multi-professionals working across organisational boundaries. A report by the Standing Medical and Nursing & Midwifery Advisory Committees*. Leeds: Department of Health, 1996a.

Department of Health. *Primary care: delivering the future*. London: HMSO, 1996b.

Department of Health. *Choice and opportunity: primary care: the future*. London: HMSO, 1996c.

Department of Health. *Planning the medical workforce. Medical Workforce Standing Advisory Committee: third report*. London, 1997.

Department of Health, Health Service Circular. *Commissioning in the new NHS – commissioning services 1999–2000*. HSC 1998/198. London: Department of Health, 1998a.

Department of Health, Health Service Circular. *Nurse prescribing: implementing the scheme across England*. HSC 1998/232. London: Department of Health, 1998b.

Department of Health, Health Service Circular. *Health improvement programmes: planning for better health and better health care*. HSC 1998/167. London: Department of Health, 1998c.

Department of Health, Health Service Circular. *Planning for health and health care. Incorporating guidance for health and local authorities on health improvement programmes, service and financial frameworks, joint investment plans and primary care investment plans.* HSC 1999/244. London: Department of Health, 1999a.

Department of Health. *Saving lives: our healthier nation.* London: TSO, 1999b.

Department of Health. *Future staffing requirements: the government's response to the Health Committee's report on future staffing requirements.* London: TSO, 1999c.

Department of Health. *Mental health national service framework: workforce planning, education and training underpinning programme. Interim report by the Workforce Action Team.* London: Department of Health, 2000a.

Department of Health. *Comprehensive critical care: a review of adult critical care services.* London: Department of Health, 2000b.

Department of Health. *National service framework for coronary heart disease.* London: Department of Health, 2000c.

Department of Health. *A health service of all the talents: developing the NHS workforce. Consultation Document on the Review of Workforce Planning 2000.* London: TSO, 2000d.

Department of Health. *Research and development for a first class service: R&D funding in the new NHS.* Leeds: Department of Health, 2000e.

Department of Health. *NHS R&D Funding. Consultation paper: NHS priorities and needs R&D funding.* London: Department of Health, 2000f.

Department of Health. *Shaping the future NHS: long term planning for hospitals and related services: consultation document on the findings of the National Beds Inquiry.* London: TSO, 2000g.

Department of Health. *Outpatient services.* National Patient Access Team. Leeds: Department of Health, 2000h.

Department of Health. *Out of hours services.* London: Department of Health, 2000i.

Department of Health. Press Release 2000/0658, 2000j.

Department of Health. *Report on Winter 1999/2000.* Millennium Executive Team. Leeds: Department of Health, 2000k.

Department of Health and NHS Management Executive. *Integrating primary and secondary health care: a paper by the NHS Management Executive.* London: NHS Management Executive, 1991.

Department of Health and Welsh Office. *A policy framework for commissioning cancer services: a report by the Expert Advisory Group on Cancer to the Chief Medical Officers of England and Wales.* London: Department of Health, 1995.

Department of Health and NHS Executive. *Patient partnership: building a collaborative strategy*. Leeds: Department of Health, 1996.

Department of Health and NHS Executive. *NHS priorities and planning guidance 1998/99*. EL(97)39. Leeds: Department of Health, 1997.

Department of Health and NHS Executive. *Additional resources in 1998–99 for 'whole systems' action to support sustained reductions in NHS waiting lists*. HSC 1998/096. Leeds: Department of Health, 1998a.

Department of Health and NHS Executive. *The new NHS 1998 reference costs*. Leeds: NHS Executive, 1998b.

Department of Health and NHS Executive. *Managing the new NHS: functions and responsibilities in the new NHS*. Undated.

Department of Health and Social Security. *The National Health Service: the future structure of the National Health Service*. London: HMSO, 1970.

Department of Health and Social Security. *Management arrangements for the reorganised National Health Service*. London: HMSO, 1972.

Department of Health and Social Security. *Priorities for health and personal social services in England. A consultative document*. London: HMSO, 1976.

Department of Health and Social Security. *The way forward*. London: HMSO, 1977.

Department of Health and Social Security. *Patients first*. London: HMSO, 1979.

Department of Health and Social Security. *Medical Manpower Steering Group Report*. London: HMSO, 1980a.

Department of Health and Social Security. *Hospital services: the future of hospital provision*. London: HMSO, 1980b.

Department of Health and Social Security. *Care in action*. London: HMSO, 1981.

Department of Health and Social Security. *Neighbourhood nursing: a focus for care: report of the Community Nursing Review*. London: HMSO, 1986.

Dixon M, Sweeney K. *The human effect in medicine: theory, research and practice*. Oxford: Radcliffe Medical Press, 2000.

Donohoe M T. Comparing generalist and specialty care. *Arch Intern Med* 1998; 158: 1596–1608.

Dowie R *et al*. A decision analytic approach to commissioning ambulance cardiac services. *Journal of Management in Medicine* 1998; 12 (2): 81–91.

Doyle L, Cameron A. Reshaping the NHS workforce: necessary changes are constrained by professional structures from the past. *BMJ* 2000; 320: 1023–4.

Ebrahim S, Redfern J. *Stroke care – a matter of chance*. London: The Stroke Association, 1999.

Edwards N. Barrier grief. *Health Service Journal* 2000; March: 28–9.

Edwards P *et al*. *Shared care: a model for clinical management*. Oxford: Radcliffe Medical Press, 1996.

Ellis B W, Johnson S. A clinical view of pathways of care in disease management. *International Journal of Health Care Quality Assurance* 1997; 10 (2): 61–6.

Exworthy M, Powell M, Mohan J. The NHS: quasi-market, quasi-hierarchy and quasi-network? *Public Money & Management* CIPFA 1999; 15–22.

Ferguson B, Sheldon T, Posnett J. *Concentration and choice in health care*. London: Financial Times Healthcare, 1997.

Ferguson T. Online patient-helpers and physicians working together: a new partnership for high quality health care. *BMJ* 2000; 321: 1129–32.

Fischer E S, Welch H G. Avoiding the unintended consequences of growth in medical care: how might more be worse? *Journal of the American Medical Association* 1999; 281 (5): 446–53.

Fox D M. *Health policies, health politics. The British and American experience 1911–1965*. Princeton, New Jersey: Princeton University Press, 1986.

Francis C M, Caruana L, Kearney P, Love M, Sutherland G R, Starkey I R, Shaw T R D, McMurray J J V. Open access echocardiography in management of heart failure in the community. *BMJ* 1995; 310: 634–6.

Franks P, Fiscella K. Primary care physicians and specialists as personal physicians: health care expenditures and mortality experience. *Journal of Family Practice* 1998; 47: 105–9.

Fries J F, Everett Koop C, Sokolov J, Beadle C E, Wright D. Beyond health promotion: reducing need and demand for medical care. *Health Affairs* 1998: 17: 70–84.

Fulop N J, Hood S, Parsons S. Does the National Health Service want hospital-at-home? *Journal of the Royal Society of Medicine* 1997; 90: 212–15.

Gardner K, Chapple A. Barriers to referral in patients with angina: qualitative study. *BMJ* 1999; 319: 418–21.

Gervas J, Perez Fernandez M, Starfield B H. Primary care, financing and gatekeeping in Western Europe. *Family Practice* 1994; 11 (3): 307–17.

Gillies R R *et al*. Conceptualising and measuring integration: findings from the Health Systems Integration Study. *Hospital & Health Services Administration* 1993; 38 (4): 467–89.

Gillis C R, Hole D J. Survival outcome of case by specialist surgeons in breast cancer: a study of 3786 patients in the West of Scotland. *BMJ* 1996; 312: 145–8.

Glasby J, Littlechild R. Fighting fires? – emergency hospital admission and the concept of prevention. *Journal of Management in Medicine* 2000; 14 (2): 109–18.

Glied S. Getting the incentives right for children. *Health Services Research* 1998; 33 (4): 1143–59.

Godfrey M, Williams T. *Referrals and admissions to the acute service: ward and intensive home treatment team*. Leeds: Nuffield Institute for Health, 1998.

Green J M, Curtis P, Price H, Renfrew M J. *Continuing to care. The organisation of midwifery services in the UK: a structured review of the evidence*. Cheshire: Books for Midwives Press, 1998.

Greenhalgh T, Herxheimer A, Isaacs A J, Beaman M, Morris J, Farrow S. Commercial partnerships in chronic disease management: proceeding with caution. *BMJ* 2000; 320: 566–8.

Gregg J, Appleton R E. Community child health: an essential specialist service for the millennium. *Lancet* 1999; 354 (Suppl II): 28–30.

Grimley Evans J. Education and debate. *BMJ* 1997; 315: 1075–7.

Grumbach K, Bodenheimer T. The organization of health care. *Journal of the American Medical Association* 1995; 273: 160–7.

Grumbach K, Selby J V, Damberg C *et al*. Resolving the gatekeeper conundrum. What patients value in primary care and referrals to specialists. *JAMA* 1999; 282: 261–6.

Guillebaud C W, chair. *Report of the Committee of Enquiry into the Cost of the National Health Service*. London: HMSO, 1956.

Gutch R. Cynics may mock, but patient empowerment changes lives. *Primary Care Report* 2000; 2 (10) 22, 24.

Hadorn D, Holmes A. The New Zealand priority criteria project. Part 1: Overview; Part 2: Coronary artery bypass graft surgery. In New B, editor. *Rationing: Talk and action in health care*. London: BMJ and King's Fund, 1997.

Hallam L, Wilkin D, Roland M, editors. *24 hour responsive health care*. Manchester: National Primary Care Research and Development Centre, 1996.

Hamblin R, Harrison A, Boyle S. *Why waiting lists grow*. Unpublished, available from AH.

Hampton J R, Gray A. The future of general medicine: lessons from an admissions ward. *Journal of the Royal College of Physicians of London* 1998; 32 (1): 39–43.

Harbison J, Massey A, Barnett L, Hodge D, Ford G A. Rapid ambulance protocol for acute stroke. *Lancet* 1999; 353: 1935.

Harries J *et al*. *Elephant problems and fixes that fail: the story of a search for new approaches to inter-agency working*. London: King's Fund, 1999.

Harrison A, Prentice S. *Acute futures*. London: King's Fund, 1996.

Harrison A. *London's health care system*. London: King's Fund, 1997.

Harrison A. *National services frameworks*. In: Klein R. *Implementing the White Paper*. London: King's Fund, 1998.

Harrison A, New B. *Access to elective care: the real way to tackle waiting lists*. London: King's Fund, 2000.

Harrison A, Dixon J. *The NHS: facing the future*. London: King's Fund, 2000.

Hart J T. The inverse care law. *Lancet* 1971; 1: 405–12.

Hart J T. Clinical and economic consequences of patients as producers. *Journal of Public Health Medicine* 1995; 17 (4): 383–6.

Haycox A, Bagust A, Walley T. Clinical guidelines – the hidden costs. *BMJ* 1999; 318: 391–3.

Health Service Management Unit. *The future healthcare workforce*. Manchester: University of Manchester, 1996.

Health Service Management Unit, University of Manchester. *The future healthcare workforce: the second report*. Bournemouth: Bournemouth University, 1999.

Hermanek P, Hohenberger W. The importance of volume in colorectal cancer surgery. *European Journal of Surgical Oncology* 1996; 22: 213–15.

Heymann T D, Culling W. The patient focused approach: a better way to run a hospital. *Journal of the Royal College of Physicians of London* 1996; 30 (2): 142–4.

Hicknan M, Drummond N, Grimshaw J. The operation of shared care for chronic disease. *Health Bulletin* 1994; 52 (2): 118–26.

Hill C, Woodcock J. *The National Health Service*. London: C Johnson, 1949.

Holman H, Lorig K. Patients as partners in managing chronic disease. *BMJ* 2000; 320: 526–7.

Holt P R. *Cost effectiveness in hospitals. Clinical services in perspective*. London: FT Pharmaceuticals, Financial Times Business, 1999.

Honigsbaum F. *The division in British medicine: a history of the separation of general practice from hospital care 1911–1968*. London: Kogan Page, 1979.

House of Commons Health Committee. *Maternity services: volume 1: second report [of the] Health Committee, together with appendices and the proceedings of the Committee*. London: HMSO, 1992.

House of Commons Health Committee. *Future NHS staffing requirements: volume 1: report and proceedings of the Committee*. London: TSO, 1999a.

House of Commons Health Committee. *Future NHS staffing requirements: volume 2: minutes of evidence and appendices*. London: TSO, 1999b.

House of Commons Select Committee on Science and Technology. *Cancer research – a fresh look. Sixth report.* London: TSO, 2000.

House of Commons Social Services Committee. *Medical education, with special reference to the number of doctors and the career structure in hospitals: volume 1. Fourth report.* London: HMSO, 1981.

House of Commons Social Services Committee. *Medical education report: follow-up.* London: HMSO, 1985.

House of Commons Welsh Affairs Committee. *Treatment centres: first report, together with the proceedings of the committee, minutes of evidence and appendices.* London: HMSO, 1995.

House of Lords. *Priorities in medical research: third report of the Select Committee on Science and Technology, session 1987–88.* London: HMSO, 1988.

Hunter D J. The changing roles of health care personnel in health and health care management. *Social Science and Medicine* 1996; 43 (5): 799–808.

Hunter D J, Fairfield G. Disease management. *BMJ* 1997; 315: 50–3.

Ibbotson K. The role of the clinical nurse specialist: a study. *Nursing Standard* 1999; 14 (9): 35–8.

Isaacs B. Is geriatrics a specialty? In: *Health care of the elderly*. London: Croom Helm, 1981.

Jarhult J. The importance of volume for outcome in cancer surgery – an overview. *European Journal of Surgical Oncology* 1996; 22: 205–10.

Jenkins C. *Personal medical services pilots: progress and prospects.* London: King's Fund, 1999.

Jenkins-Clarke S *et al. Skill mix in primary care: a study of the interface between the general practitioner and other members of the primary health care team: a final report.* York: University of York, 1997.

Jervis R. *System effects: complexity in political and social life.* New Jersey: Princeton University Press, 1997.

Johnson S, editor. *Pathways of care*. Oxford: Blackwell Science, 1997.

Johnston K, Sussex J, editors. *Surgical research and development in the NHS – promotion, management and evaluation.* London: Office of Health Economics, 1997.

Joint Consultants Committee. *Organisation of acute general hospital services.* London: JCC, 1999.

Kalra L, Evans A, Perez I, Knapp M, Donaldson N, Swift C G. Alternative strategies for stroke care: a prospective randomised controlled trial. *Lancet* 2000; 356: 894–9.

Kendrick S, Frame S, Povey C. Beds occupied by emergency patients: long term trends in patterns of short-term fluctuation in Scotland. *Health Bulletin* 1997; 55 (3): 167–75.

Kerr D, editor. The future of general medicine. *Journal of the Royal College of Physicians of London* 1998; 32 (March/April): 2.

Kerrigan D D, Brown S R, Hutchinson G H. Open access gastroscopy: too much to swallow? *BMJ* 1990; 300: 374–6.

King M, Petchey R. *Building bridges: integrating primary and secondary care for people with HIV/AIDS*. Bristol: Policy Press, 1997.

King's Fund. *Memorandum of evidence*. In: House of Commons Health Committee. *Planning the NHS Workforce, Vol II. Appendix* 68. London: TSO, 1999.

King's Fund. *NHS priorities and needs funding. King's Fund response to consultation paper*. London: King's Fund, 2000.

King's Fund Centre. *Hospital at home: the coming revolution*. London: King's Fund Centre, 1989.

King's Fund Management College. *Integrated approaches to child health care: a submission to the Health Select Committee: the results of a seminar held at the King's Fund, hosted by the Royal Victoria Infirmary NHS Trust, facilitated by the King's Fund Management College*. London: King's Fund, 1996.

Kirkness B, editor. *Putting patients first: the emerging role of patients in the provision of healthcare*. London: Association of the British Pharmaceutical Industry, 1996.

Kisely S, Green J, Howell K. Pathways to orthodontic care. *Journal of Public Health Medicine* 1997; 19 (2): 148–55.

Klein R, editor. *Implementing the White Paper: pitfalls and opportunities*. London: King's Fund, 1998.

Kohn L T, Corrigan J M, Donaldson M S, editors. *To err is human: building a safer health system*. Washington, DC: National Academy Press, 2000.

Kurowski B. Cancer carve outs, specialty networks and disease management: a review of their evolution, effectiveness and prognosis. *American Journal of Managed Care*, 1997; Vol. 4, special issue.

Langhorne P, Dennis M, editors. *Stroke units: an evidence based approach*. London: BMJ, 1998.

Layton A, Moss F, Morgan G. Mapping out the patient's journey: experiences of developing pathways of care. *Quality in Health Care* 1998; 7: 530–6.

Lecky F, Woodford M, Yates D W. Trends in trauma care in England and Wales 1989–97. *Lancet* 2000; 355: 1771–5.

Le Grand J, Mays N, Mulligan J, editors. *Learning from the NHS internal market*. London: King's Fund, 1998.

Leutz W N, Greenlick M R, Capitman J A. Integrating acute and long-term care. *Health Affairs* 1994; 13 (4): 58–74.

Leutz W N. Five laws for integrating medical and social services: lessons from the United States and the United Kingdom. *Milbank Quarterly* 1999: 77 (1): 77–110.

Levenson R, Joule N. *Improving people's lives. The agenda for people with long-term medical conditions*. London: LMCA, 1999.

Levy M L *et al. Shared care for asthma*. Oxford: Isis Medical Media, 1997.

Lewis R, Jenkins C, Gillam S. *Personal medical services pilots in London. Rewriting the Red Book*. London: King's Fund, 1999.

Loefler I J P. More on specialization. *Surgery* 1998; 16 (2): i.

Loefler I J P. The renaissance of general surgery. *BMJ* 2000; 320: 436–8.

Loeser J D, Melzack R. Pain: an overview. *Lancet* 1999; 353: 1607–9.

London Implementation Group. *Plastics and burns: report of an independent review of specialist services in London*. London: HMSO, 1993.

Long Term Medical Conditions Alliance. *Improving lives – proposals for change*. London: LMCA, 1999.

Luce J M, Byyny R L. The evolution of medical specialism. *Perspectives in Biology and Medicine* 1979; 22: 377–89.

MACA. *First national GP survey of mental health in primary care*. London: MACA, 1999.

McClenahan J, Mumford P. *A long slow road ahead in improving cancer services*. Mimeo unpublished.

McColl E, Hutchinson A. An agenda for change in referral: consensus from general practice. *British Journal of General Practice* 1994; 44: 157–62.

McCormack B, Ford P. The contribution of expert gerontological nursing. *Nursing Standard* 1999; 13: 42–5.

McKee M, Black N. Hours of work of junior hospital doctors: is there a solution? *Journal of Management in Medicine* 1991; 5: 40–54.

Mackenzie W J M. *Power and responsibility in health care: the National Health Service as a political institution*. London: Oxford University Press for the Nuffield Provincial Hospitals Trust, 1979.

McKeown T. *Medicine in modern society*. London: George Allen & Unwin Ltd, 1965.

McLachlan G, McKeown T. *Medical history and medical care: a symposium of perspectives*. London: Oxford University Press for the Nuffield Provincial Hospitals Trust, 1971.

McLachlan G, editor. *Positions, movements and directions in health services research: the papers and proceedings of a meeting held at Hertford College, Oxford, 1974*. London: Oxford University Press for Nuffield Provincial Hospitals Trust, 1974.

McLachlan G, editor. *Five years after: a review of health care research management after Rothschild*. Oxford: Oxford University Press, 1978.

McLachlan G. A *fresh look at policies for health service research and its relevance to management*. London: Nuffield Provincial Hospitals Trust, 1985.

McLachlan G. *What price quality?* London: Nuffield Provincial Hospitals Trust, 1991.

McLachlan G. *What price quality? The NHS in review*. London: Nuffield Provincial Hospitals Trust, 1990.

Maggs-Rapport F, Kinnersley P, Owen P. In-house referral: changing general practitioners' roles in the referral of patients to secondary care. *Social Science and Medicine* 1998; 46 (1): 131–6.

Mainous III A G, Baker R, Parker S G. Hospitalists for the NHS? *Journal of the Royal Society of Medicine* 2000; 93: 504–6.

Malcolm L. Service management: a New Zealand model for shifting the balance from hospital to community care. *International Journal of Health Planning and Management* 1991; 6: 23–35.

Malcolm L. Service management: an epidemiological model of health services organization. *Journal of Health Administration Education* 1993; 11 (4): 563–74.

Malcolm L. Primary health care and the hospital: incompatible organisational concepts. *Social Science and Medicine* 1994; 39 (4): 455–8.

Marks L. *Seamless care or patchwork quilt? discharging patients from acute hospital care*. London: King's Fund Institute, 1994.

Marsh G, Renfrew M, editors. *Community-based maternity care*. Oxford: Oxford University Press, 1999.

Maynard A, Walker A. Managing the medical workforce: time for improvements? *Health Policy* 1995; 31: 1–16.

Mays N *et al*. *What were the achievements of total purchasing in their first year and how can they be explained*. London: King's Fund, 1998.

Medical Manpower Steering Group. *Report*. London: DHSS, August 1980.

Medical Workforce Standing Advisory Committee. *Planning the medical workforce. Medical Workforce Standing Advisory Committee: third report*. Department of Health: London, 1997.

Memel D. Chronic disease or physical disability? The role of the general practitioner. *British Journal of General Practice*, 1996; 46: 109–13.

Merrison A, chair. *Report of the Committee of Inquiry into the Regulation of the Medical Profession*. Cm 6018. London: HMSO, 1975.

Merrison A, chair. *Report of Royal Commission on the National Health Service*. Cm 7615. London: HMSO, 1979.

Millard P H. A case for the development of departments of gerocomy in all district general hospitals: discussion paper. *Journal of the Royal Society of Medicine* 1991; 84: 731–3.

Millard P H, McClean I S. *Modelling hospital resource use: a different approach to the planning and control of health care systems*. London: Royal Society of Medicine Press, 1994.

Millard P H, McClean I S, editors. *Go with the flow: a systems approach to healthcare planning*. London: Royal Society of Medicine Press, 1996.

Millard P H, Christodoulou G. Measuring and modelling patient flow. *British Journal of Health Care Management* 2000; 6 (10): 463–8.

Miller A B, To T, Baines C J, Wall C. Canadian National Breast Screening Study 2: 13-year results of a randomized trial in women aged 50–59 years. *Journal of the National Cancer Institute* 2000; 92 (18): 1490–9.

Miller R H. Health system integration: a means to an end. *Health Affairs* 1996; 15 (2): 92–106.

Ministry of Health. *The Dawson report on the future provision of medical and allied services 1920: an interim report to the Minister of Health*. Consultative Council on Medical and Allied Services. London: King Edward's Hospital Fund for London, 1950.

Ministry of Health. *National Health Service: a hospital plan for England and Wales*. Cm 1604. London: HMSO, 1962.

Ministry of Health. *National Health Service: the administrative structure of the medical and related services in England and Wales*. London: HMSO, 1968.

Ministry of Health. *The functions of the district general hospital*. London: HMSO, 1969.

Ministry of Health. *The future structure of the National Health Service*. London: HMSO, 1970.

Ministry of Health. *National Health Service reorganisation*. Cm 5055. London: HMSO, 1972.

Ministry of Health and Department of Health for Scotland. *A national health service*. London: HMSO, 1944.

Monaghan S, Davidson J, Bainton D. *Freeing the dragon: new opportunities to improve the health of the Welsh people*. London: The Nuffield Trust, 1999.

Moscovice I, Wellever A, Christianson J *et al*. Understanding integrated rural health networks. *The Milbank Quarterly* 1997; 75 (4): 563–88.

Muir Gray J A. Postmodern medicine. *Lancet* 1999; 354: 1550–3.

Mullan F. The 'Mona Lisa' of health policy: primary care at home and abroad. *Health Affairs* 1998; 17 (2): 118–26.

Mulligan J-A. *Breast cancer: why are deaths falling?* London: King's Fund, 2000a.

Mulligan J-A. *Estimating the contribution of health care to health.* London: King's Fund, 2000b.

Munro J. *et al. Evaluation of NHS Direct first wave sites: first interim report to the Department of Health.* Sheffield: University of Sheffield, School of Health and Related Research, Medical Care Research Unit, 1998.

Munro J. *et al. Evaluation of NHS Direct first wave sites: second interim report to the Department of Health.* Sheffield: University of Sheffield, School of Health and Related Research, Medical Care Research Unit, 2000.

Murray J. *Cleft lip and/or palate: report of a CSAG committee.* London: TSO, 1998.

National Assembly for Wales. *Emergency pressures planning guidance winter 2000/01.* Cardiff: 2000.

National Assembly for Wales. *Health: clinical pathways.* Cardiff: 2000.

National Association of Health Authorities and Trusts. *Reinventing healthcare.* Birmingham: NAHAT, 1993.

National Association of Health Authorities and Trusts. *Closer to home: healthcare in the 21st century.* Birmingham: NAHAT, 1994.

Nazarko L. Improving discharge: the role of the discharge co-ordinator. *Nursing Standard* 1998; 12 (49): 35–7.

New B, Klein R. *Rationing: talk and action in health care.* London: BMJ and King's Fund, 1997.

New B. The NHS: what business is it in? In: Harrison A, editor. *Health Care UK 1997/98.* London: King's Fund, 1998.

Newchurch Working Paper. *New strategies for acute hospitals.* Newchurch, 1999.

NHS Centre for Reviews and Dissemination. *Relationship between volume and quality of health care: a review of the literature 1995.* York: University of York NHS CRD, 1995.

NHS Confederation. *Changing hospitals: unpacking secondary care.* London: NHS Confederation, 2000.

NHS Confederation. *A vision for primary care: applying the modernisation approach.* London: NHS Confederation, 2000.

NHS Management Executive. *Integrating primary and secondary health care.* London: NHS Management Excutive, 1991a.

NHS Management Executive. *Managing resource management projects: practical experience*. London: Department of Health, 1991b.

NHS Executive. *The patient's progress: towards a better service*. London: HMSO, 1994.

NHS Executive. *Specialist Workforce Advisory Group, annual report for 1995/96*. 1996.

NHS Executive. *Commissioning in the new NHS*. HSC 1998/198. 1998a.

NHS Executive. *The NHS home healthcare guide*. Leeds: NHSE, 1998b.

NHS Executive. *Changing childbirth development projects*. London: NHS Executive, 1998c.

NHS Executive. *Additional resources in 1998–99 for 'whole systems' action to support sustained reductions in NHS waiting lists*. Leeds: NHS Executive, 1998d.

NHS Executive. *Service delivery and organisation programme*. London: NHS Executive, 2000a.

NHS Executive. *Millenium Executive Team report on winter 1999/2000*. London: NHS Executive, 2000b.

NHS Executive. *The NHS cancer plan: a plan for investment, a plan for reform*. London: NHS Executive, 2000c.

NHS Executive, Anglia and Oxford Region. *Opportunities in emergency health care: summary report from the Anglia and Oxford emergency health care project*. London: Arena Communications and Design, 1995.

NHS Executive, Anglia and Oxford Region. *Opportunities in intermediate care: summary report from the Anglia and Oxford intermediate care project*. Milton Keynes: NHS Executive Anglia & Oxford, 1997.

NHS Executive, Institute of Health Services Management, NHS Confederation. *In the public interest: developing a strategy for public participation in the NHS*. London: Department of Health, 1998.

NHS Executive, North Thames. *The right team for the job*. London: NHS Executive, 1997.

NHS Executive, North Thames. *The workforce project: a report of two behavioural simulations exploring the interaction between health care and education and training pressures on the clinical workforce*. London: NHS Executive North Thames and Office for Public Management, 1997.

NHS Executive, South Thames. *Review of cervical screening services at Kent and Canterbury Hospitals NHS Trust*. London: NHS Executive South Thames, 1997.

NHS Trust Federation. *Specialist trusts – the key issues*. London: NHS Trust Federation, 1997.

NHS Wales. *Access and excellence: acute health services in Wales*. Cardiff: NHS Wales, 2000.

Newchurch & Company Limited. *New strategies for acute hospitals: developing a strategic direction*. London: Newchurch & Company Limited, 1999.

Nichol J, Turner J, Dixon S. *The cost-effectiveness of the Regional Trauma System in the North West Midlands: final report to the Department of Health*. Sheffield: SCHARR, 1995.

Nichol J, Munro J. Systems for emergency care. Integrating the components is the challenge. *BMJ* 2000; 320: 955–6.

Nocon A, Baldwin S. *Trends in rehabilitation policy: a review of the literature*. London: King's Fund, 1998.

Nuffield Provincial Hospitals Trust. *Specialized futures: essays in honour of Sir George Godber* GCB. Series on Problems and Progress in Medical Care. Essays on current research. London: Oxford University Press, 1975.

Office for Public Management. *The workforce project: a report of two behavioural simulations exploring the interaction between health care and education and training pressures on the clinical workforce*. Leeds: Department of Health, 1997.

Oni O A O. Hospital management in the 1990s: fundholding consultants? *Journal of Management in Medicine* 1994; 8: 64–70.

Oni O A O. *Who should run the health service?* Oxford: Radcliffe Medical Press, 1996.

Organisation for Economic Co-operation and Development. *New directions in health care policy*. OECD: Paris, 1995.

Owen D, MP, editor. *A unified health service*. Oxford: Pergamon Press, 1968.

Packwood T, Keen J, Buxton M. *Hospitals in transition: the resource management experiment*. Milton Keynes: Open University Press, 1991.

Packwood T, Keen J, Buxton M. Process and structure: resource management and the development of sub-unit organisational structure. *Health Services Management Research* 1992; 5 (1): 66–76.

Parry N, Parry J. *The rise of the medical profession*. London: Croom Helm, 1976.

Peck E, Parker E. Mental health in the NHS: policy and practice 1979–98. *Journal of Mental Health* 1998; 7 (3): 241–59.

Peckham R, Smith R, editors. *Scientific basis of health service*. London: BMJ, 1996.

Pencheon D. Matching demand and supply fairly and efficiently. *BMJ* 1998; 316 (7145): 1665–7.

Perkins B B. Shaping institution-based specialism: early twentieth-century economic organization of medicine. *Social History of Medicine* 1997; 10 (3): 419–35.

Pratt J, Plamping D, Gordon P. *Partnership: fit for purpose?* London: King's Fund, 1998.

Pratt J, Gordon P, Plamping D. *Working whole systems. Putting theory into practice in organisations*. London: King's Fund, 1999.

Preston C, Cheater F, Baker R, Hearnshaw H. Left in limbo: patients' views on care across the primary/secondary interface. *Quality in Health Care* 1999; 8: 16–21.

Pringle M L K. *11,000 seven-year-olds: first report of the National Child Development Study (1958 Cohort): submitted to the Central Advisory Council for Education (England)*. London: Longmans, 1966.

Pristave R J, Becker S, Gutierrez L. Development of provider networks for specific diseases. *Journal of Health Care Finance* 1995; 22 (2): 27–41.

Public Audit Forum. *Implications for audit of the modernising government agenda*. London: Public Audit Forum, 1999.

Rafferty A M. *The politics of nursing knowledge*. London: Routledge, 1996.

Rafferty A M, Robinson J, Elkan R, editors. *Nursing history and the politics of welfare*. London: Routledge, 1997.

Reeves D *et al*. *Direct referral systems for hearing aid provision*. London: HMSO, 1994.

Report of the Committee on Child Health Services. *Fit for the future*. London: HMSO, 1976.

Richardson G, Maynard A. *Fewers doctors? More nurses? A review of the knowledge base of doctor–nurse substitution – Discussion Paper 135*. York: University of York Centre for Health Economics, Health Economics Consortium, NHS Centre for Reviews & Dissemination, 1995.

Rivett G. *From cradle to grave: fifty years of the NHS*. London: King's Fund, 1998.

Robert G, Stevens A. Should general practitioners refer patients directly to physical therapists? *British Journal of General Practice* 1997: 47 (418): 314–18.

Robinson J C. The changing boundaries of the American hospital. *Milbank Quarterly* 1994; 72 (2): 259–75.

Robinson J C, Casalino L P. Vertical integration and organizational networks in health care. *Health Affairs* 1996; 15 (1): 7–22.

Robinson J C. *The corporate practice of medicine: competition and innovation in health care*. Berkeley: University of California Press, 1999.

Rogers A, Entwistle V, Pencheon D. A patient-led NHS: managing demand at the interface between lay and primary care. *BMJ* 1998; 316 (7147): 1816–19.

Rogers R, Hassell K, Nicolas G. *Demanding patients? Analysing the use of primary care*. Buckingham: Open University Press, 1999.

Roland M, Coulter A, editors. *Hospital referrals*. Oxford: Oxford University Press, 1992.

Rosen G. Medical thought and the rise of specialism. *CIBA Symposia* 1949; 11: 1126–34.

Royal College of General Practitioners. *The front line of the Health Service*. London: Royal College of General Practitioners, 1987.

Royal College of Physicians. *Future patterns of care by general and specialist physicians. Meeting the needs of adult patients in the UK*. London: Royal College of Physicians of London, 1996.

Royal College of Physicians. *Hospital doctors under pressure: new roles for the health care workforce*. London: Royal College of Physicians, 2000.

Royal College of Physicians and Royal College of Psychiatrists. *The psychological care of medical patients: recognition of need and service provision*. London: Royal College of Physicians, 1995.

Royal College of Physicians of England. *The consultant physician: responding to change*. London: Royal College of Physicians, 1996.

Royal College of Surgeons. *Report of the Working Party on Head Injuries*. London: Royal College of Surgeons, 1986.

Royal College of Surgeons of England. *The provision of emergency surgical services: an organisational framework*. London: Royal College of Surgeons, 1997.

Royal College of Surgeons of England and British Orthopaedic Association. *Better care for the severely injured*. London: Royal College of Surgeons of England, 2000.

Royal Commission on Medical Education. *Report [of the] Royal Commission on Medical Education 1965–68*. Cm 3569. London: HMSO, 1968.

Royal Commission on the National Health Service. *Doctor manpower 1975–2000: alternative forecasts and their resource implications. Research Paper Number 4*. London: HMSO, 1978.

Royal Commission on the National Health Service. *Royal Commission on the National Health Service: Report*. London: HMSO, 1979.

Royal Pharmaceutical Society of Great Britain and British Medical Association. *Teamworking in primary healthcare: realising shared aims in patient care*. London: RPSGA and BMA, 2000.

Ryan B, Culham L. *Fragmented vision: survey of low vision services in the UK*. London: RNIB, Moorfields NHS Trust, 1999.

Salisbury C, Dale J, Hallam L, editors. *24-hour primary care*. Oxford: Radcliffe Medical Press Ltd, 1999.

Salmon S *et al*. Telemedicine use in two nurse-led minor injuries units. *Journal of Telemedicine and Telecare* 2000; 6 (Suppl.1) S1: 43–5.

Sanazaro P J. Historical discontinuity, hospitals and health services. In: McLachlan G, McKeown G, editors. *Medical history and medical care: a symposium of perspectives*. London: Nuffield Provincial Hospitals Trust, 1971.

Schellevis F G. *Chronic diseases in general practice. Comorbidity in quality of care*. Ph.D thesis available from author. University of Nijmegen, 1993.

Scottish Office. *Acute services review*. Edinburgh: TSO, 1998.

Scottish Office. *Introduction of managed clinical networks within the NHS in Scotland*. NHS MEL (1999) 10. Edinburgh: 1999.

Secretaries of State for Health. *Working for patients*. Cm. 555. London: HMSO, 1989.

Secretaries of State for Social Services, Wales, Northern Ireland and Scotland. *Primary health care: an agenda for discussion*. London: HMSO, 1986.

Secretary of State for Health. *Primary health care: an agenda for discussion*. Cm. 9771. London: HMSO, 1986.

Secretary of State for Health. *A service with ambitions*. London: HMSO, 1996.

Secretary of State for Health. *The New NHS: modern, dependable*. Cm. 3807. London: TSO, 1997.

Secretary of State for Health. *Saving lives: our healthier nation*. London: TSO, 1999.

Secretary of State for Health. *The NHS Plan: a plan for investment, a plan for reform*. London: TSO, 2000.

Sefrin P, Weidringer J W. History of emergency medicine in Germany. *Journal of Clinical Anaesthesiology* 1991; 3: 245–7.

Semple-Piggot C, Shapiro J, Smith J. *Holding a mirror to the primary care led NHS: comparative gatekeeping in Holland, Denmark and the UK*. Birmingham: HSMC, 1997.

Shi L. Primary care, specialty care, and life chances. *International Journal of Health Services* 1994; 24 (3): 431–58.

Shi L. Balancing primary versus specialty care. *Journal of the Royal Society of Medicine* 1995; 88: 428–32.

Shortell S M, Gillies R R, Anderson D A. The new world of managed care: creating organized delivery systems. *Health Affairs* 1994; 13 (5): 46–64.

Shortell S M, Gillies R R, Devers K J. Reinventing the American hospital. *Milbank Quarterly* 1995; 73 (2): 131–59.

Shortell S M, Kaluzny A D. *Essentials of health care management*. Albany, NY: Delmar Publishers, 1997.

Simpson J, Smith R. Why healthcare systems need medical managers. *BMJ* 1997; 314: 1636–7.

Silvester K. Chaos, the enemy of quality. *Clinician in Management* 1997; 6 (5): 9–13.

South-East Thames Regional Health Authority. *Shaping the future: a review of acute services*. Bexhill-on-Sea: SETRHA, 1991.

Standing Medical Advisory Group. *Future patterns of medical care*. London: SMAC, 1997.

Standing Medical and Nursing & Midwifery Advisory Committees. *In the patient's interest. Multi-professional working across organisational boundaries*. London: Department of Health, 1996.

Starfield B. Is primary care essential? *Lancet* 1994; 344: 1129–33.

Starfield B, *Primary care: balancing health needs, services and technology*. Oxford: OUP, 1998.

Steel R J C. The influence of surgeon case volume on site specific cancer. *European Journal of Surgical Oncology* 1996; 22: 211–13.

Stevens R. *Medical practice in modern England: the impact of specialization and state medicine*. New Haven: Yale University Press, 1966.

Stevens R. The changing idea of a medical specialty. *Transactions and Studies of the Royal College of Physicians of Philadelphia 2*. 1980: 159–77.

Stevens R. *In sickness and in wealth. American hospitals in the twentieth century*. USA: Basic Books Inc, 1989.

Stowe, Sir Kenneth. *On caring for the National Health*. London: Nuffield Provincial Hospitals Trust, 1989.

Stroke Association. *Stroke. National tragedy, national priority: an agenda for action in stroke prevention, treatment and care*. London: The Stroke Association, 1997.

Taylor D. *Hospital at home: the coming revolution*. London: King's Fund Centre, 1989.

Taylor I. Super-specialisation in cancer surgery – How beneficial? *Surgery* 1997; 15 (5): ii.

Taylor T R, Gordon M J. Developing a unitary model of the clinical management process. In: Sheldon M *et. al. Decision-making in general practice*. Basingstoke: Macmillan, 1985.

Thomas D, Cooper L, Cooper J, Taylor D, Robb A. Direct fast track admission to a coronary care unit. *Journal of the Royal College of Physicians of London* 1997; 31: 188–91.

Tomlinson, Sir Bernard, chair. *Report of the inquiry into London's health service, medical education and research*. London: HMSO, 1992.

van Raak A, Paulus A, van Merode F, Mur-Veeman I. Integrated care management: applying control theory to networks. *Journal of Management in Medicine* 1999; 13 (6): 390–404.

van Weel C, Knottnerus J A. Evidence-based interventions and comprehensive treatment. *Lancet* 1999; 353: 916–18.

Vaughan B, Lathlean J. *Intermediate care: models in practice*. London: King's Fund, 1999.

Vincent J-L, Thijs L, Cerny V. Critical care in Europe. *International Perspectives on Critical Care* 1997; 13 (2): 245–54.

Vogel R L, Ackermann R J. Is primary care physician supply correlated with health outcomes? *International Journal of Health Services* 1998; 28 (1): 183–96.

Von Korff M, Gruman J, Schaefer J, Curry J, Wagner E H. Collaborative management of chronic illness. *Annals of Internal Medicine* 1997; 127 (12): 1097–1103.

Wade D T, de Jong B A. Recent advances in rehabilitation. *BMJ* 2000; 320: 1385–8.

Wagner E H, Austin B T, Von Korff M. Organizing care for patients with chronic illness. *Milbank Quarterly* 2000; 74: 4.

Wagner E H. The role of patient care teams in chronic disease management. *BMJ* 2000; 320: 569–71.

Wall P. *Pain: the science of suffering*. London: Weidenfeld & Nicholson, 1999.

Walsh M. *Models and critical pathways in clinical nursing: conceptual frameworks for care planning*. London: Bailliere Tindall, 1999.

Warner M, Riley C. *Closer to home: healthcare in the 21st century*. Birmingham: NAHAT, 1994.

Warner M, Longley M, Gould E *et al. Healthcare futures 2010*. Pontypridd: Welsh Institute for Health and Social Care, 1998.

Weddell J M, Beresford S A A. *Planning for stroke patients. A four-year descriptive study of home and hospital care*. London: HMSO, 1979.

Weed L J. New connections between medical knowledge and patient care. *BMJ* 1997; 315 (26 July 1997).

Weiner C L. *The elusive quest: accountability in hospitals*. New York: Aldine de Gruyter, 2000.

Welsh Office. *NHS Wales: putting patients first*. London: TSO, 1998.

Wilson J, editor. *Integrated care management: the path to success?* Oxford: Butterworth-Heinemann, 1997.

Wolfe C, Rudd T, Beech R, editors. *Stroke services and research: an overview, with recommendations for future research*. London: The Stroke Association, 1997.

Wood B. *Patient power?* Buckingham: Open University Press, 2000.